1984

A Resource Allocation Model for Child Survival

A Resource Allocation Model for Child Survival

Howard Barnum
University of Michigan

Robin Barlow
University of Michigan

Luis Fajardo
Universidad del Valle, Cali, Colombia

Alberto Pradilla
World Health Organization

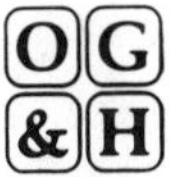
Oelgeschlager, Gunn & Hain, Publishers, Inc.,
Cambridge, Massachusetts

International Standard Book Number: 0–89946–052–6

Library of Congress Catalog Card Number: 80–17933

Printed in the United States of America

Library of Congress Cataloging in Publication Data

Main entry under title:

A Resource allocation model for child survival.

"This project was carried out by the Center for
Research on Economic Development, University of
Michigan, under a contract from the United States Agency
for International Development, Office of Health.
U.S.A.I.D. project no. 931–11–590–260; U.S.A.I.D.
contract no. AID/ta-C-1358."
Includes index.
1. Underdeveloped areas—Child health services—Cost effectiveness—Mathematical models. 2. Underdeveloped areas—Children—Mortality—Mathematical models. 3. Underdeveloped areas—Infants—Mortality—Mathematical models. I. Barnum, Howard Nelch. II. Michigan. University. Center for Research on Economic Development. III. United States. Agency for International Development. Office of Health.
RJ101.R44 362.1'9892 80–17933
ISBN 0–89946–052–6

This project was carried out by the Center for Research on Economic Development, University of Michigan, under a contract from the United States Agency for International Development, Office of Health.

Contents

List of Figures

List of Tables

Preface

This study develops a mathematical optimization model designed to provide policymakers with an analytical framework to facilitate the efficient allocation of resources to programs intended to reduce the rate of child mortality. The model is used to provide a direct assessment of health interventions to raise the probability of child survival in a specific locality, but the approach presented has general application to an analysis of the cost effectiveness of alternative health programs. At the core of the approach is a multiple disease morbidity-mortality model that allows the estimation of the disease incidence and mortality levels that result from a given health intervention policy. Major features of the model include the consideration of disease interaction, the distinction between preventive activities affecting morbidity and curative activities affecting case fatality rates, the separation of the early childhood period into age subgroups with distinct morbidity characteristics, and the distinction between program usage and program availability.

The diseases chosen for the analysis account for at least 75 percent of childhood mortality and have well-known and obvious potential interventions. Low birth weight, birth trauma, infections, and tetanus are considered for the neonatal age group; and malnutrition, diarrhea, lower respiratory diseases, and immunizable childhood diseases are considered for the infant and toddler age groups. General categories of interventions considered include prenatal care, immunizations, nutritional programs, water and sanitation, promotional programs, and institutional care.

The parameters that determine the impact of the health interventions on morbidity, case fatality, and usage are specified from the results of subjective estimates derived from a survey of health professionals with clinical, research, and field experience. Survey results indicate that the greatest impacts on morbidity are expected from promotional, water, sanitation, and nutritional programs. Further, the survey indicates that significant interdisease causal effects are expected to exist between diarrhea and malnutrition. However, the relative impacts of the interventions and the degree of disease interaction cannot be used separately to guide policy; the impacts must be considered in tandem with costs to determine the most effective allocation of resources.

Costs and baseline data were assembled for a hypothetical community resembling as closely as practical a low-income urban area of Cali, Colombia. The highest cost activities are inpatient care and institutional deliveries. Nutritional activities are moderately expensive. The least expensive activities per unit are health promotion, latrines, well-baby clinics, and prenatal iron supplements.

Before turning to the optimization analysis the characteristics of the model were explored in a series of simulations. Simulations with the model using baseline intervention levels and the subjective specification of impact parameters produce a pattern of mortality by cause of death that corresponds to the patterns for comparable communities observed in the Pan American Health Organization study directed by Puffer and Serrano. Other simulations confirmed the importance of promoting program usage. Simulations revealed that a general feature of the model is the diminished marginal cost effectiveness of any given activity as the level of other activities increases. The cross impact between the effectiveness of one activity and the level of another make it particularly difficult to examine the cost effectiveness of separate activities out of the context of other associated health activities.

The optimization model applied in this study makes it possible to consider the joint cost effectiveness of a set of health activities. Alternative degrees of resource scarcity are considered in the optimization experiments. At low levels of resources, the activities selected for emphasis are health promotion, water and sanitation, and well-baby clinics. These activities act to promote breast feeding and to lower diarrhea and, through disease interaction, to lower malnutrition. Outpatient treatment for neonatal children and prenatal tetanus immunization are also chosen for resource-poor communities.

As the community resources increase to middle levels, nutritional activities, immunizations, and outpatient care for the older age groups are adopted. Prenatal care activities and the general coverage of the programs selected at the lower resource levels are also increased. At the highest resource levels considered, an upgrading of activities occurs as inpatient care replaces outpatient care and home water and toilets replace public fountains and latrines.

The reduction in child mortality with the optimum use of resources is dramatic at low resource levels and diminishes as resources become more abundant. Similarly the value of the constraining resources falls as the general level of resources increases. Registered nurse time and peso budgets are found to be the binding constraints, and a high proportion of available auxiliary nurse time is used in most of the optimization experiments. A possible implication is that manpower training programs should place more emphasis on the training of nurses.

Acknowledgments

One of the rewards of directing this study has been the opportunity to work with the many people who have made contributions at various stages. I have especially appreciated the opportunity to know and work with my collaborators—Robin Barlow, Luis Fajardo, and Alberto Pradilla. Robin Barlow has collaborated in the design of the general morbidity–mortality model presented in Chapter 3. Luis Fajardo and Alberto Pradilla collaborated in the selection of intervention activities, diseases, and other characteristics of the specific model and in the design and conduct of the survey of professional opinion. I am also grateful for the assistance and outstanding competence of Richard Parsons, who did much of the computer coding, selected the optimization program used in the analysis, and spent many nights carrying out the computer simulations and optimization experiments.

A sizable debt is owed to Peter Heller who identified this area as important and feasible for research and who spent considerable time over the period of a year negotiating the contract proposal and setting up the initial contacts between the Center for Research on Economic Development, Universidad del Valle, and the Colombian ministry of health that made the project possible.

An important debt is also owed the participants in the survey of professional opinion without whom the project could not have been completed:

Drs. Alfredo Aguirre, Edgar Cobo, William Cutting, Jean-Pierre Habicht, A. Herrera, James Koopman, David Morley, Hernando Rey, Jaime Rodriguez, Alfonso Santemaria, F. M. Shattock, A. Tafur, Ronald Wilson, and Joe D. Wray. Their participation allowed the specification of the model's parameters, but it is pointed out that the final specification does not necessarily reflect the opinion of any one participant and participation does not imply approval of the interpretation of project results given in the study.

We are fortunate to have had the encouragement, advice, and help of Gildardo Agudelo, Elliot Berg, Edgar Ariza-Nino, Stanley Garn, Thomas Hyslop, James Koopman, George Simmons, and Irving Taylor. Dr. Jaime Rodriguez, former director of the PRIMOPS project in Cali, Colombia, was especially generous in providing help at several stages of the project.

An important factor contributing to the project has been the pleasant and stimulating professional environment maintained at the Center for Research on Economic Development under the former director Elliot Berg and present director Robin Barlow. Administrative and accounting assistance was provided cheerfully and expertly by Sherry Cogswell and Jane McCormick. Secretarial matters were smoothly coordinated in Ann Arbor by Jayne Owen and in Colombia by Magda Hernandez. Numerous tables and equations made the manuscript especially difficult to type and we appreciate the efforts of Linda Burnett Schultz, Denise Castilloux, Judith Dubermann, Lori Rankin, and Jeane Walkowski. Chris Augustyniak, Donna Alexander, and Rand Baldwin provided bibliographical and data assistance.

We appreciate the cooperation of the government of Colombia, especially of Dr. Raul Orejuela Bueno, minister of health and Dr. Ricardo Galan. We also appreciate the help given by the Fundacion para la Educacion Superior, especially Dr. Alex Cobo, in the administration of the project in Colombia. Finally it is noted that the design of the model and interpretation of results do not necessarily reflect the policies of the government of Colombia, the Fundacion para la Educacion Superior, or the United States Agency for International Development.

Howard Barnum
Ann Arbor

Chapter 1

Introduction and Summary

High rates of infant and toddler mortality are one of the heavier burdens borne by the populations of the less-developed world. The factors underlying the relatively low probability of child survival are intricately interwoven and are not amenable to piecemeal curative or preventive medical or health policies. Yet throughout the less-developed world, efforts at raising the probability of child survival are fragmented across different operating agencies. Rarely are the minimal resources devoted to primary health care carefully marshalled to deal efficiently with the most pressing health and medical problems of the population. One partial explanation for the inadequacy of current efforts has been the failure of policy analysts to determine an integrated and cost-effective approach to the alleviation of community health problems that underlie high infant mortality rates.

The objective of the project described here is to provide policymakers with an analytical framework that will facilitate the efficient allocation of resources to programs intended to reduce the rate of child mortality. The project is used to provide direct assessment of health interventions designed to raise the probability of child survival in a hypothetical community modeled after a specific locality, but the techniques developed are intended to have general application to an analysis of the cost effectiveness of alternative health programs.

An important belief underlying the analysis is that direct interventions are a practicable means of improving the rate of child survival in less-developed countries. The potential improvement in mortality rates is demonstrated by a comparison of health statistics in developed countries with data from less-developed countries. Life expectancy at birth throughout the developing world averages about two-thirds of the level of the developed countries. A substantial part of this difference is explained by the dramatic differences in infant and childhood mortality between the less-developed and more-developed countries. In the poorest regions of the world over 10 percent of all children born die within the first year of life. In contrast, in Western Europe and the United States less than 1.5 percent of all children born die within the first year of life. Between the high rates of childhood mortality in developing countries and the low rates in developed countries lie large differences in demographic and economic conditions affecting child survival, as well as differences in the level of community infrastructure and health services. Economic development is obviously the major requirement for the ultimate achievement of a fully satisfactory nutritional and health status. But development is a slow process and there is growing evidence that the use of direct health and environmental interventions can bring about a substantial improvement in health status, especially in infancy and early childhood before development has occurred. The technical feasibility of alternative interventions has been demonstrated in numerous projects involving, for instance, nutritional programs, improvement of water quantity and quality, provision of preventive services, and provision of curative clinical care.

In spite of technical feasibility, resource constraints restrict the adoption of projects and for this reason health programs must also be examined with respect to economic feasibility. Bilateral, multilateral, and private donor agencies as well as domestic governments have markedly increased the availability of resources for health projects over the last decade. But in spite of these increased resources, the total still falls far short of what would be required to adopt all the alternative interventions that might be considered. The binding resource constraints are not always funds; they may involve, depending on the time and place, financial restrictions, limited administrative capacity, shortage of skilled personnel, or limits on the size of physical facilities. Often programs from alternative donors compete for the same set of resources so that, for example, a prenatal-care program funded by one international donor may use scarce registered nurse administrative time also needed for a child-immunization program funded by another donor or domestic government agency. As a result, the effectiveness of both programs is cut by faulty administration. Thus, as the example illustrates, health programs need to be coordinated and a careful choice must be made among alternative programs competing for the limited resources available.

From one point of view the choice may not appear difficult. It can be argued that health conditions in many developing countries are so poor that almost any improvement that might be considered by a knowledgeable and responsible health planner will bring about a dramatic improvement in health status. To a certain extent our findings provide some reinforcement of this view since we found that very poor countries can expect a large decrease in mortality with any of the nutritional or preventive care interventions considered here.

But on closer inspection of the problem, it is apparent that the choice may actually be more difficult. Although a dramatic improvement in the number of children born who survive through early childhood may be obtained with any of the alternatives considered, the improvement per unit of resources allocated differs significantly among the alternatives. The best health program will, of course, consist of the set of interventions bringing about the greatest improvement in child survival for a given level of resource expenditures. If any other set of interventions is chosen there will be an unnecessary waste of resources and an unnecessarily high level of childhood mortality. In a high-income country the penalty for an incorrect choice of resources is likely to be low. But in a poor country, with a high initial level of child mortality and an acute scarcity of resources, the penalty for a suboptimum choice of interventions is likely to be high. If scarce money, manpower, and facilities are to be used to the best effect, then interventions must be chosen carefully with tandem concern for program effects and costs.

POLICY ISSUES

The choice of interventions raises several policy issues that are broader in scope than the detailed examination of the cost effectiveness of individual health measures. These are issues of emphasis on broad classes of interventions, program organization, and choice of target population subgroups. Although our analysis is designed to answer questions about the optimum use of resources for specific interventions, the results also provide tentative answers to questions that arise in considering several of the broader issues. Among these are the following:

Curative Versus Preventive Care

Is curative care cost effective? The use of large-scale physical facilities (hospitals and clinics) to provide capital intensive curative care for limited population subgroups has fallen into justified disrepute. It is clearly recognized that these facilities do not represent a cost effective use of resources. The continued construction of large-scale curative facilities is attributable to political processes and decisions and not to an erroneous assessment of the cost effectiveness of these programs on the part of health planners. But the possible use of smaller-scale curative facilities, especially for outpatient care, remains an important ongoing question. Low-technology therapies, such as oral rehydration of diarrhea patients, can be administered at the level of small health clinics and health posts. The question of cost effectiveness of low technology curative care versus preventive care remains of interest.

A closely related question is that of mode of birth delivery. The demand for institutional delivery has in many areas caused a substantial allocation of health resources to delivery clinics. Many health planners feel that midwife-attended home deliveries would allow a more efficient distribution of health resources in resource-poor communities. The model applied here allows a comparison of alternative modes of birth delivery and also a comparison of curative versus preventive use.

Promotion Versus Services

How should resources be divided between health promotion and the actual provision of services? The question of access versus usage remains important for both preventive care and curative care programs. In the promotional programs considered here, health workers with only a low level of education visit households and track the health status of children and women, encourage the consistent use of breast feeding throughout the infant period, and convey information about health services. Recent experiments with health promotion programs in Candelaria, Colombia, and elsewhere demonstrate that the effectiveness of health services can be raised through early detection of pregnancy, tracking of child growth progress, and identification of high-risk children.

Water and Sanitation Versus Health Services

Are water and sanitary interventions cost effective in comparison with direct health services? The cost effectiveness of water and sanitation is expected to vary greatly over communities depending on the community's location and density. In the water and sanitation programs examined here, community population density is high, water resources are available, and an existing urban water and sewage infrastructure provides economies of scale so that the cost of extending the programs to the study community is relatively low. In this respect the results may not be of broader application. In general, however, water and sanitation programs do not rely heavily on continuing inputs of skilled manpower. Thus, if the important constraint on health programs is the availability of skilled manpower, water and sanitation programs may be competitive alternatives to other health programs.

Population Target Groups

Even though the ultimate objective of the policies considered is the lowering of child mortality, the appropriate population targets are not obvious. Is it the prenatal, neonatal, infant, or early childhood period that should receive the most attention? The answer depends not only on the relative mortality in each population group but on the relative costs and effects of interventions aimed at the mortality problems of each group.

A second problem in the choice of population group is that of screening for high-risk targets. Is it cheaper to first incur the cost of examinations and tests for screening before providing treatment to a selected high-risk group, or to omit screening and provide treatment to a larger group without attempting to identify high-risk individuals? For example, is it more cost effective to provide nutritional supplements to all pregnant women or to first screen pregnant women by risk group and then provide nutritional supplements only to those evaluated as high risks of having low-birth-weight children? The answer is not obvious without analysis. It depends on the costs of screening, the proportion of pregnant women who are high risks, the cost of the nutritional programs, and the relative effectiveness of the alternative nutritional programs.

Resource Constraints

What are the binding constraints? Interventions use differing proportions of different resources. Some health activities draw heavily on the use of physical facilities, others draw heavily on the time of skilled personnel, still others draw heavily on budgeted funds. Are the effective restrictions on the adoption of health programs to improve child survival primarily limits in budgets, personnel, or physical facilities? The answer to this question has important implications for long-term manpower planning, building programs, and budgeting. The resource allocation model developed here allows the identification of constraining resources and estimates the benefits to be derived from additional resources.

ORGANIZATION OF RESEARCH

A schematic presentation of the general optimization problem can be used to explain the natural order and partitioning of the research tasks involved in the child mortality project. Figure 1–1 presents a schema for

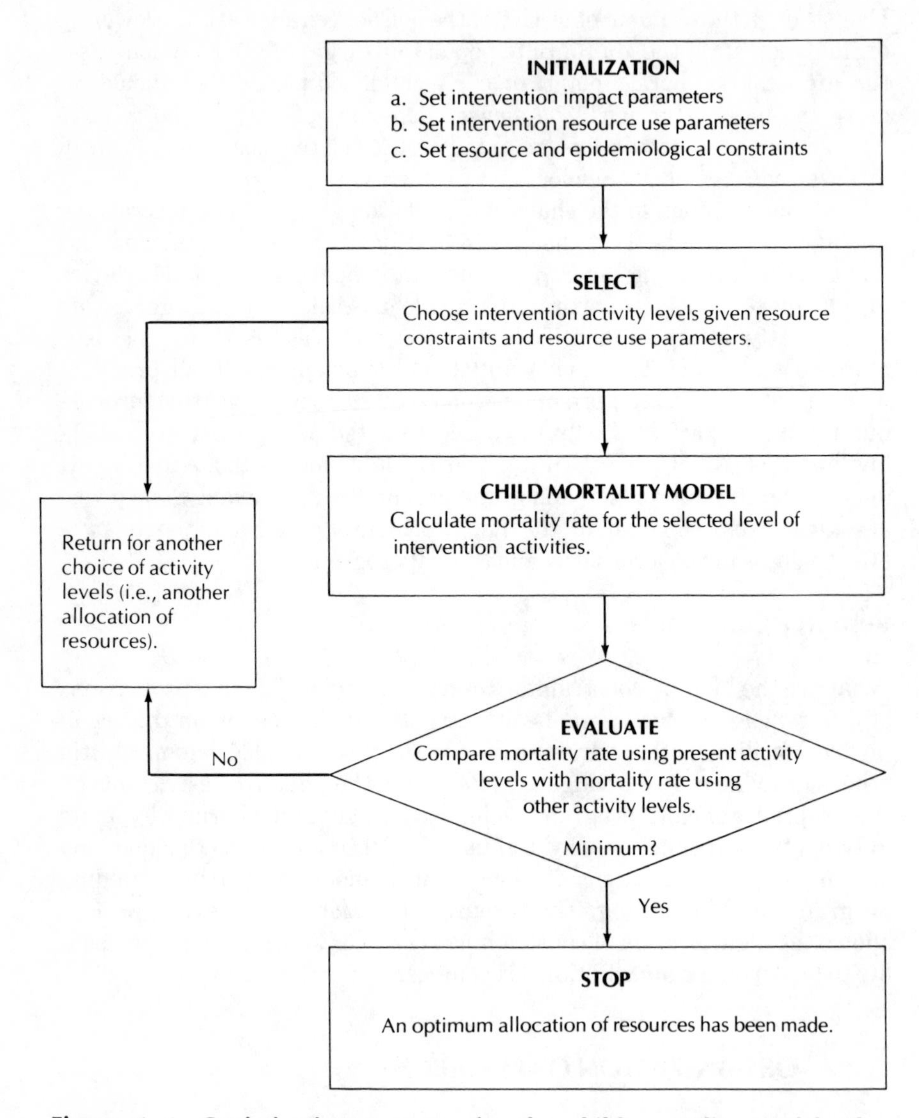

Figure 1–1. Optimization program for the child mortality model. The objective is to achieve the lowest possible level of infant mortality given the available resources and possible health activities.

the organization of an optimization program designed to allocate given resources among competing health interventions to achieve the lowest possible level of child mortality. Although the child mortality problem involves a nonlinear optimization program, the approach used to obtain an optimum solution parallels that used in a linear optimization program. First, the epidemiological characteristics of the population, the availability of resources, and the effectiveness of various health interventions are set. Second, a choice of intervention activity levels lying within the resource constraints for the locality under analysis is made.[a] Third, the level of the objective, the rate of child mortality, is calculated given the choice of intervention activities. Finally, the second two steps are repeated and an optimization algorithm is used to determine whether a minimum mortality rate has been reached or whether a further selection of activity levels should be made.

The optimization problem thus results in the following four distinct phases of the project.

1. The development of a model of the process by which infants and toddlers are exposed to mortality risks and of the way in which alternative strategies may alter the process.
2. Specification of the parameters of the model through a survey of medical and public health professionals regarding the impact of alternative health interventions on infant mortality.
3. Estimation of the cost of alternative health interventions, an assessment of available resources, and the specification of baseline epidemiological and demographic data.
4. The application of simulation and nonlinear optimization procedures to determine the set of interventions that are most cost effective in raising the probability of child survival, given the design of the model and the estimated effectiveness of interventions.

THE CHILD MORTALITY MODEL

The design of a model of the child mortality process proceeded in two stages. In the first stage, the algebraic and logical relationships for a general model of morbidity and mortality were developed. The goal at this stage was to derive an algebraically logical and appropriate model that is sufficiently simple to be amenable to the repeated calculation of a solution needed in the optimization program, yet sufficiently complete to include

[a] More precisely, the optimization technique used assigns a penalty to the objective function if the resource constraints are exceeded. A heuristic discussion of the optimization method is given later.

essential medical relationships and provide potential answers to the policy questions raised earlier. In Chapter 2 the model is first set forth for two diseases and then extended to cover an indefinite number of morbidity categories.

In the second stage the general model was specified to conform to the relationships between diseases and interventions relevant to child mortality. The major consideration of this part of the research was to insure the medical accuracy of the model's relationships and to choose practical health interventions that might actually be considered by a rapidly developing country with high levels of child mortality. Major features of the model include: (1) the use of interactive simultaneous equations to model the causes of death in a setting of multiple diseases; (2) the clear distinction between preventive activities affecting morbidity and curative activities affecting case fatality rates; and (3) the distinction between program usage and availability. These features allow an analysis of the policy issues discussed earlier. Chapter 3 presents a summary of the specific child mortality model, including interventions and disease categories, that forms the basis of the simulation program used in the analysis.

The diseases included in the model underlie, or are associated with, three-quarters or more of childhood mortality in most developing countries. Low birth weight, birth trauma, infections and neonatal tetanus are involved in the preponderance of mortality occurring in the first four weeks following birth; and malnutrition, diarrhea, lower respiratory infections and immunizable diseases account for over 80 percent of infant and toddler mortality. Broadly classified, the interventions to be evaluated include prenatal care, nutritional programs, immunizations, promotional programs, institutional care and improved water and sanitation.

The general structure of the model can be summarized here. The central feature is a set of disease-specific morbidity rates calculated as functions of the level of *use* of health interventions and also, simultaneously, functions of the level of other morbidity rates. The disease-specific morbidity rates are used, following the procedures described in Chapter 2, to calculate the proportion of the population with given combinations of diseases. Case fatality rates for each disease combination are calculated as functions of the *use* of curative services. Finally the mortality rates are computed as the product of morbidity and case fatality rates and the overall mortality rate is obtained by summation of the mortality rates for the individual disease combinations.

Separate submodels are specified for the neonatal, infant, and early childhood (toddler) age groups. The mortality rates calculated in younger age groups are used to calculate the number of survivors moving into the next older age group. Starting from a given number of births and given levels of interventions the number of survivors from one age group to the next is calculated in sequence. The overall objective in the resource allocation is to maximize the number of children surviving from birth through the end of the oldest age group included in the model.[b]

By including interactions between diseases, the child mortality model allows for indirect as well as direct effects of interventions. An example is provided by the relation between programs primarily attacking nutritional deficiency and those attacking child diarrhea, and the further relation of both of these categories of programs to mortality from childhood communicable diseases for which immunizations exist ("immunizable diseases"). Recent research has examined the interrelationship between diarrhea and malnutrition, and it seems clear that chronic diarrhea reduces the quantity of nutrients absorbed and leads to a deterioration in nutritional status. At the same time a plausible argument is made that children with low nutritional status are more susceptible to diarrhea. It also seems clear that the case fatality rates for children suffering from immunizable diseases are higher for malnourished children than for children of normal nutritional status. It is apparent, then, that water and sanitation programs may have effects that are greater than just their direct effect on diarrhea morbidity; the programs can also act indirectly to improve nutritional status and reduce fatality rates from immunizable diseases. Similarly, nutritional programs act indirectly to reduce mortality from both diarrhea and immunizable diseases. The relative cost effectiveness of nutritional, water, and immunization programs depends not only on their relative costs and their direct affects on malnutrition, diarrhea, and immunizable diseases, respectively, but also on their indirect effects transferred through disease interaction.

By allowing for interactions between diseases and also by distinguishing between case fatality rates for different disease combinations, the model includes the subtle, indirect effects of interventions and thus provides a more balanced assessment of the cost effectiveness of alternative interventions than could be obtained by considering the obvious direct effects alone.

SPECIFICATION OF IMPACT PARAMETERS

The calculation of the morbidity and fatality rates for selected levels of intervention activities and the socioeconomic characteristics of

[b] Other objectives, such as minimization of morbidity rather than mortality, could have been defined. Also, an objective function combining weighted levels of morbidity and/or mortality could have been used. The weights could vary with age group or disease. However, the use of alternative objective functions would have carried the study too far afield. We preferred to restrict the objective function to the definition given above (maximization of the number of survivors from birth through early childhood) rather than direct the study to an analysis of the complex, philosophical questions brought forth by considering alternative objectives.

the population requires an estimate of the impact of these variables. Several problems arise in the specification of the quantitative relationships between the various policy interventions and the probability of contracting and surviving different disease problems. Perhaps the most accurate specification would involve the statistical analysis of morbidity and fatality data resulting from alternative interventions and socioeconomic conditions. But for many of the interventions and disease categories, the technological and physiological relationships are not fully understood, and even where the theoretical relationships are explicit, no suitable body of data exist that would allow their empirical specification. It is clear that providing the full set of technological parameters through the normal process of medical research might delay any comprehensive analysis of alternative policy interventions until the distant future.

A survey of health practitioners was chosen as an alternative, practical means of specifying the intervention effects. In spite of the dearth of explicit theoretical information, a sufficient wealth of practical experience and knowledge exists to allow the use of "Bayesian" or "Delphi" techniques to estimate the needed quantitative relationships at a level of accuracy adequate for policy analysis. It is obvious that policy choices are often made using government policymakers' subjective evaluations of the impact of health policies. The use of a subjective survey to specify the parameters of a model such as the present one allows the subjective evaluations of health planners to be combined with information about costs to facilitate the choice of the most cost-effective policies.

A survey procedure and a set of survey questions sufficient to provide point estimates of the policy coefficients of the model were developed. The survey respondents included health professionals with clinical, research, and field experience. Chapter 5 summarizes the survey results and discusses the derivation of the policy parameters of the model. Briefly, the survey results indicate that the greatest impacts on morbidity are expected from promotional, water, sanitation, and nutritional programs. Further, the survey indicates that significant interdisease causal effects are expected to exist between diarrhea and malnutrition. However, the relative impacts of the interventions and the degree of disease interaction cannot be used separately to guide policy; the impacts must be considered jointly with costs to determine the most effective allocation of resources.

COSTS AND BASELINE DATA

The need for cost information and baseline data requires the selection of a community for analysis. After consideration of several sites, it was decided to locate the analysis in Cali, Colombia, in the area of the

Programa de Investigacion en Modelos de Prestacion de Servicios de Salud (PRIMOPS) project, which is currently being carried out by the Universidad del Valle and Tulane University under a contract with the United States Agency for International Development (AID). An important advantage of this site was that a preliminary morbidity and demographic survey, which can provide baseline data, was carried out at the inception of the PRIMOPS project. A second advantage was that an objective of the PRIMOPS project is to obtain information about the cost of interventions similar to those being considered here. Both the baseline morbidity data and the cost data are preliminary and approximate and for this reason the specific quantitative results of the analysis are tentative.

Nevertheless the data are adequate for the purpose of illustrating the feasibility and possible applicability of the child mortality model. It is important to note, however, that the optimum intervention levels chosen in the analysis are sensitive to the relative resource costs of the competing interventions. In this study, the highest cost activities are inpatient care and institutional deliveries. Nutritional activities are moderately expensive. The least expensive activities are health promotion, latrines, well-baby clinics, and prenatal iron supplements. Chapter 4 presents the baseline population and morbidity data and Chapter 6 discusses the estimation of program costs.

APPLICATION OF THE MODEL

The model can be applied in either single simulations or in optimization experiments involving repeated simulation. Given a specification of the impact and cost parameters, simulation with the model produces estimates of the morbidity and mortality outcomes and the rate of survival from birth through early childhood implied by a given choice of intervention policies that maximize the probability of child survival.

Before turning to the optimization analysis, simulations are used to explore the model's characteristics, and also to check the operational consistency of the model against observed data. With regard to consistency, simulations with the model using baseline intervention levels and the subjective specification of impact parameters produce a pattern of mortality by cause of death that corresponds to the patterns for comparable communities observed in the Pan American Health Organization study directed by Puffer and Serrano.[1] With regard to the model's characteristics, simulations with the model demonstrate the importance of disease interdependence, the importance of usage promotion, and the decline in cost of curative care with increases in preventive health activities. Simulations also illustrate the dramatic returns, in terms of lowered mortality, to increased health resources in resource-poor communities, and the decline in returns to health resources in communities with greater resources. Chapter 7 discusses the results of simulations with the model. A general feature of the model is the diminished marginal cost effectiveness of any given activity as the level of other activities increases. The cross impact between the effectiveness of one activity and the level of another make it particularly difficult to examine the cost effectiveness of separate activities out of the context of other associated health activities. The optimization model applied here makes it possible to consider the joint cost effectiveness of a set of health activities.

Alternative degrees of resource scarcity are considered in the optimization experiments. The results reveal a definite pattern in the optimum choice of activities as resources become more abundant. At low levels of resources, the activities selected for emphasis are health promotion, water and sanitation (public fountains, latrines, and covered sewage), and inexpensive preventive clinic care. These activities act to promote breast feeding and to lower diarrhea and, through disease interaction, to lower malnutrition. Outpatient treatment for neonatal children and prenatal tetanus immunization are also chosen for resource-poor communities.

As the community resources increase to middle levels, nutritional activities, immunizations, and outpatient care for the older age groups are adopted. Prenatal care activities and the general coverage of the programs selected at the lower resource levels are also increased. At the highest resource levels considered, an upgrading of activities occurs as inpatient care replaces outpatient care, and home water and toilets replace public fountains and latrines. Chapter 8 discusses some limitations of the optimization procedure and presents the results of the optimization analysis.

For the modeled community, answers to the policy questions raised earlier can be summarized briefly. With regard to curative care, it is found that inpatient care and hospital deliveries are cost ineffective, and not adopted by the optimization program until community resources reach high levels. But it is found that neonatal and infant outpatient care are chosen at low to middle resource levels.

Promotion, both the use of home visits by promoter health workers and the use of mass media, is given strong emphasis by the allocation model. Simulations demonstrate that an important reason for the emphasis is the reduction in diarrhea and increase in nutritional status that is assumed (according to the subjective estimates given by respondents) to accompany the promotion of breast feeding and hygienic education related to neonatal and infant diarrhea. The simulations also suggest that other important effects of the health promoter at low resource levels are to encourage the use of prenatal tetanus immunization and the use of neonatal outpatient services.

Low-technology water and sanitation interventions play an important role at low resource levels. As noted earlier, this is partly attributable to the relatively low monetary cost of the programs and the fact that they do not draw on skilled personnel time. The effectiveness of the programs is enhanced by the fact that they are not age group specific and have strong effects on diarrhea in all age groups.

Looking at the question of target age groups, no clear pattern of emphasis on any age appears. The interventions chosen would provide a mix of coverage over all age groups and the prenatal period. The use of examinations for screening before treatment of iron or nutritional deficiencies in women of childbearing age or pregnant women is not demonstrated to be cost effective until middle resource levels. Similarly screening and institutional deliveries for women with high risk of low birth weight or birth trauma is not shown to be cost effective until high resource levels.

Finally, with regard to resource constraints, the optimization experiments indicate that the reduction in child mortality with the optimum use of resources is dramatic at low resource levels and diminishes as resources become more abundant. Similarly, the value of the constraining resources falls as the general level of resources increases. Registered nurse time and financial budgets are found to be the binding constraints, and a high proportion of available auxiliary nurse time is used in most of the optimization experiments. An implication is that manpower-training programs should place more emphasis on the training of nurses.

The mathematical optimization model developed here is intended as an example of a general approach to the analyses of the cost effectiveness of health projects to reduce child mortality. But the specific results of the application carried out cannot be extrapolated directly to other communities. Before other projects can be analyzed in the framework provided by this model, the intervention impacts, costs, and baseline data for the specific problem must be assembled. Also, the diseases chosen for inclusion in the study may differ for other communities. In addition, the specific functional forms and relationships between activities contained in the present model are only some of many possibilities. Other forms and estimation procedures need to be explored as multiple disease optimization models are developed further.

NOTE

1. Ruth Puffer and Carlos Serrano, eds., *Patterns of Mortality in Childhood*, Pan American Health Organization, Scientific Publication No. 262, Washington, D.C., 1973.

Chapter 2

The Basic Mortality Model

INTRODUCTION

The core of the optimization program is the child mortality model used to calculate the mortality rate that results from the epidemiological characteristics of the population and the choice of intervention activities. The model derives complexity and nonlinearity from the characteristics of the morbidity process. But in spite of the apparent complexity, a closer inspection of the model will reveal that the logical, if not the algebraic, relationships are forthright and intuitively clear. It can be argued that for a practical application the size of the model should be increased; the degree of aggregation of the disease categories and the broad definitions used for the intervention tasks are both aspects that might allow a fruitful expansion of the model with sufficient time and funds. But given the lack of a precedent for a model such as this—previous optimization models have dealt with only one disease [1] or with an even greater level of aggregation [2] —the project's overriding objective, which is to develop a framework or technique for policy analysis, is best served by the level of aggregation used here. The model is large enough to contain many of the essential characteristics to be met with in modeling multiple disease processes but small enough to be tractable.

Salient features of the model include the use of interactive simultaneous equations to model the multiple disease causes of death, the clear distinction between preventive activities affecting morbidity and curative activities affecting case fatality rates, separation of the early childhood period into age subgroups with distinct morbidity characteristics, and the use of equation forms that represent, as appropriate, increasing, constant, and decreasing returns to additional health services. Further, the optimization program distinguishes between program usage (which an economist might view as the demand side of the market for health services) and program availability (which can be viewed as supply), and operates in such a manner as to set intervention levels that will not exceed usage demand.

SYNOPSIS OF THE MODEL

The details are elaborated elsewhere but Figure 2–1 is sufficient to gain an overview of the model and illustrate some of these features. The basic relationship, shown toward the bottom of the diagram, is the calculation of mortality rates as the product of morbidity (the morbidity rate measures the prevalence of disease in the reference population) and case fatality (the fatality rates measure the incidence of death in the diseased population). Although not shown in the diagram, separate morbidity and case fatality rates are derived for each age group and an overall mortality rate is then obtained by an appropriate summation over all disease categories.

Usage Versus Availability

The boxes at the top of the diagram represent the choice of intervention activities flowing from the selection part of the optimization program. These are conveniently partitioned into mass media and other health promotional activities, clinical activities, immunizations, water and sanitation, and nutritional activities. The level of activities, originally measured in the resource allocation part of the optimization program in terms of an absolute number of visits or other appropriate units, is recalculated as a percent of the eligible population given the demographic and epidemiological characteristics of the population as represented in the box on the right-hand side of the diagram. For some of the interventions, such as water and sanitation, this yields program availability directly. Other interventions, such as mass media, act together with socioeconomic characteristics to determine the level of program usage. Still other interventions, such as health promoters who visit the household, provide services and encourage program use.

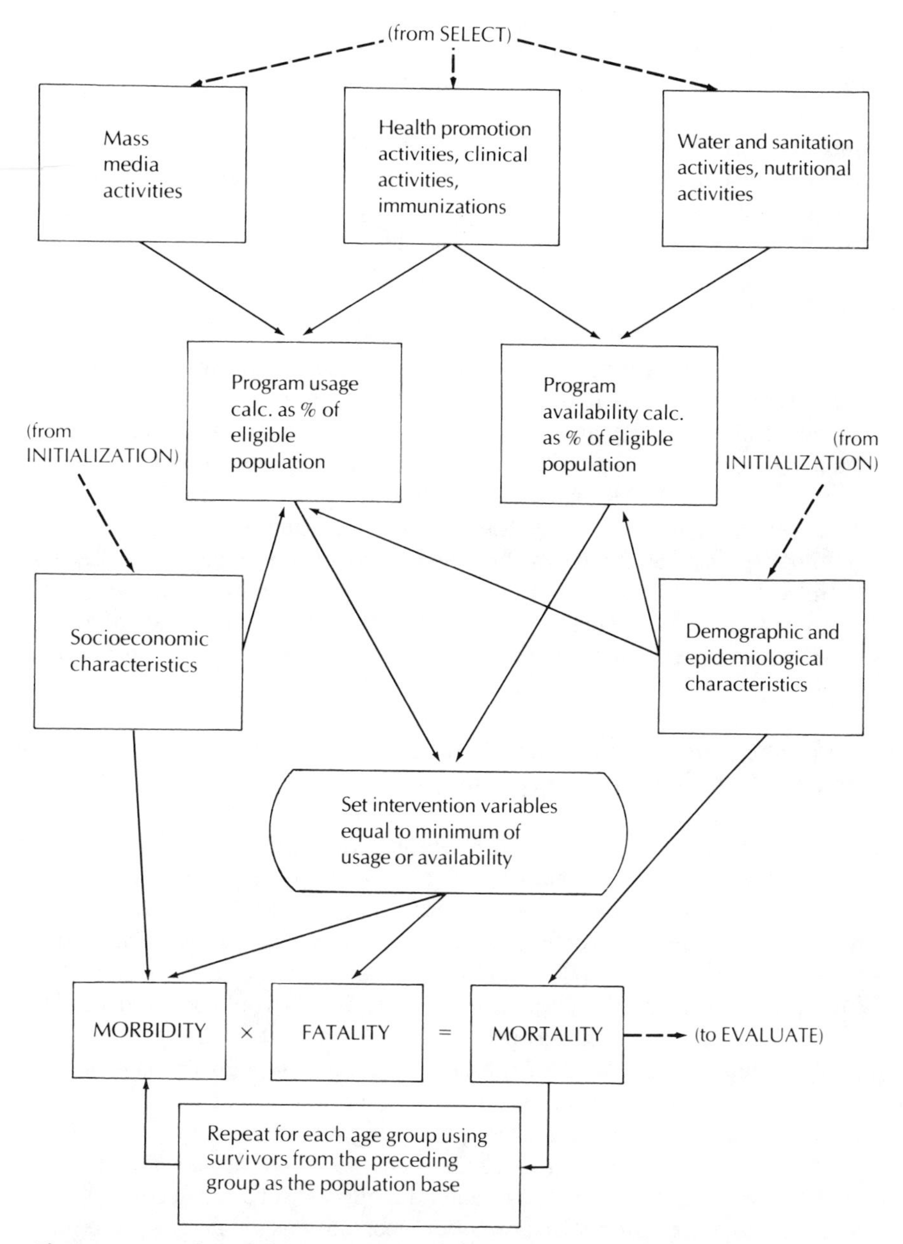

Figure 2–1. The child mortality model. This is an exploded view of the third box down in the optimization flow diagram (Figure 1–1).

Because a program must not only be available but also used in order to be effective, the model selects the minimum of usage or availability, expressed as a percent of the eligible population, to be used as the *effective* level of intervention activities in the determination of morbidity and case fatality rates. Thus, for example, if clinic capacity is 70 percent, but it is calculated that only 60 percent of the eligible population uses clinics, the morbidity and fatality rates would be calculated using 60 percent as the effective level of the clinical interventions. On the other hand, if program usage would be 100 percent, but the available capacity is only 70 percent, the calculation of morbidity and fatality rates is based on the 70-percent figure.

Age Groups

Given the effective level of intervention activities and the socioeconomic characteristics of the population, and estimates of the impact of these variables on morbidity and fatality rates, a mortality rate is calculated for each age group. Because the survivors from each age group become the population base for the next older age group, the age specific mortality rates for younger ages affect the flow of population into the box labeled "demographic characteristics" for older age groups. Repeating the process outlined in Figure 2–1 over all age groups considered in the model allows the derivation of an overall mortality rate for a baseline number of births over the first sixty months of life and for a given selection of intervention levels.

An Example of the Allocational Tradeoff Between Interventions Effecting Usage and Availability

The mortality rate thus calculated becomes one reference point (used in the diamond labeled "evaluate" in Figure 1–1) allowing the generation of an optimum resource allocation. For example, consider the equilibration of usage and availability: If an initial allocation of resources to health promotional activities leads to a low participation rate and slack capacity in intervention activities such as clinical services, this would be discovered in subsequent runs through the optimization program. It would be discovered in the evaluation segment of the program, through algorithms dictating the procedure for experimenting with intervention choices, that when resources were taken from usage-promoting activities and given to clinic activities, mortality would increase (because of decreased use of clinic services when needed), but that when resources were taken from clinical activities and used for health promotion, mortality would decrease (because of an increased use of clinic services and a reduction of slack capacity).

Similar examples can be constructed to illustrate other tradeoffs of interest, such as the tradeoff between inpatient care, which affects case fatality rates, and interventions such as water and sanitation, primarily affecting morbidity rates. In actuality, the program treats all these problems jointly and considers the simultaneous tradeoff of all interventions viewed as choice variables, although the design of the program permits some interventions to be preset at given levels and allows a restricted search over a subset of interventions of interest for particular problems.

Marginal Versus Joint Morbidity Rates

Figure 2–2 presents a detail of the calculation of the mortality rates. The diagram is intended to emphasize that the morbidity rates, that is, the marginal disease rates, are derived from functions analogous to marginal probability functions. These functions do not necessarily generate mutually exclusive rates, but instead generate the incidence of given diseases including cases where other diseases are present as well as less complicated disease states. Using these functions and a set of assumptions regarding the degree of independence between diseases, together with a set of probability relationships, mutually exclusive joint disease rates are generated. These rates can be used to calculate the distribution of the population among the disease states representing the various possible combinations of the individual diseases considered. Fatality rates for each of the mutually exclusive joint disease states are then used to calculate the state-specific mortality rate. The overall mortality rate is obtained by summing over all disease states.

By generating the morbidity structure of the model from marginal disease functions rather than directly through the use of separate functions for each of the mutually exclusive disease states, the number of parameters needed to specify the model is substantially reduced. Whereas n structural equations[a] are needed for a model of n diseases if the model is specified using marginal morbidity rates, $2^n - 1$ equations would be needed to specify the model directly at the level of the mutually exclusive disease states. In addition, the specification of the model at the level of the marginal disease rates has several other advantages that are brought out in the following discussion.

[a] The structural equations give an algebraic formulation of the model in terms of relationships that have a direct interpretation. The information contained in the equations describes the relationships between diseases and the impact of interventions and socioeconomic variables on disease incidence.

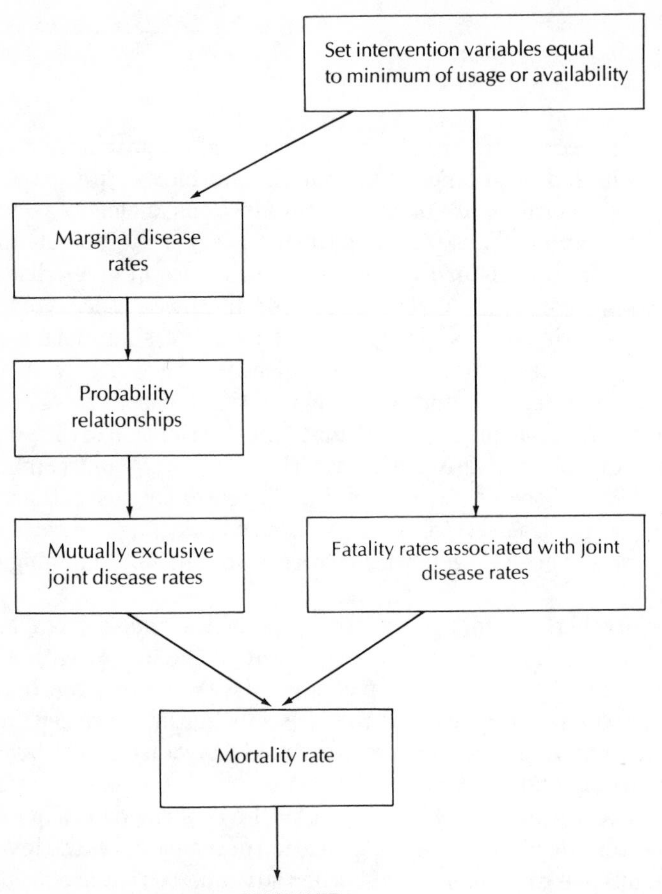

Figure 2–2. The child mortality model: detail showing calculation of mortality rates. In general it is not possible to go from a marginal distribution to a joint distribution without knowledge of the kind and degree of relationships among variables. Here we assume all diseases are independent except where an interaction is noted by the connecting arrows in Figure 3–1.

REDUCING MORTALITY WHEN DISEASES ARE INTERDEPENDENT

Comparatively little work has been done on the modeling of interdependent diseases. A recent study by Correa is typical. In developing a series of models for use in health planning, he explicitly assumes that no interdependence exists on the grounds that "fortunately, when the plan refers to short time periods, this interdependence is not likely to be important."[3] But it is not difficult to argue that interdependence might well be quite important, even in the short run. A few examples of the phenomenon can be given from the area of childhood diseases:

Gastro-enteritis leads to malnutrition, and vice versa, both conditions being major causes of child mortality in low-income countries.[4]

Measles often causes respiratory problems.[5]

Malaria produces a general debilitation, and increases the death rate from a variety of respiratory and digestive diseases.[6]

The purpose of this section is to describe a simple approach that allows for this kind of interdependence. First, some features of existing mortality risk models (which do not allow for interdependence) are reviewed. Next, a general approach to incorporating interdependence is outlined. A specific model based on two interdependent diseases is then developed, with some numerical illustrations.

Existing Models of Competing Risks

Suppose that in a population of a given age the general death rate (from all causes) is 20 percent. The death rate from a certain specific disease is 5 percent. That disease is then eliminated. What happens to the general death rate? This question is of obvious interest for our study.

One approach to this question says that the answer will definitely exceed 15 percent. This is the theory of competing risks, which points out that some of the 5 percent who would have died from the eliminated disease will now die from some other cause (during the period in question). Several models of competing risks have been developed, all of them based on mutually exclusive combination disease states. For example, refer to the models of Chiang[7] and Kimball.[8]

Interdependence has not typically been allowed for in models of competing risks. When one disease is eliminated, it is essentially assumed that the probability of catching any other disease is unaffected. With this assumption Chiang[9] derives the following formulation for answering our opening question about death rates:[b]

$$p_2' = 1 - (1 - p_1 - p_2)^{p_2/(p_1+p_2)}$$

where p_1 = probability of death from Disease 1 (later eliminated)

p_2 = probability of death from all other causes, before elimination of Disease 1.

p_2' = probability of death from all other causes, after elimination of Disease 1.

Using our numbers, $p_1 = 0.05$ and $p_2 = 0.15$. Chiang's model therefore predicts that the general death rate after the elimination of Disease 1 (that is, p_2') will be 0.154.

Kimball offers a contrasting model based on what he terms a "multinomial approach."[10] Still assuming independence of risks, he derives the following formulation for the general death rate after the elimination of Disease 1:

$$p_2' = p_2(1 - p_1)$$

With our numbers for p_1 and p_2, p_2' equals 0.158, which differs from Chiang's prediction.

In a comment on Kimball's contribution, Chiang recognizes the importance of interdependence between causes of death, and suggests that a proper method of allowing for interdependence is to specify probabilities of morbidity as well as of mortality. Models of competing risks have been deficient in not specifying morbidity rates:

> We must recognize the fact that the death of an individual is usually preceded by an illness (condition, disorder). It is not realistic to speak of a person's chance of dying from tuberculosis when he is not even affected with the disease. Also competition of risks of death depends on the health condition of an individual: a person affected with a disease (say, cardiovascular-renal (CVR) disease) probably has a probability of dying of a second disease different from a person who is not affected with CVR. Therefore, a mortality study is incomplete unless illness is taken into consideration.[11]

[b] The notation follows that used in the version of Chiang's model presented by Kimball, "Models for Estimation of Competing Risks."

Following Chiang's suggestion, in the next section we develop an alternative approach to an analysis of mortality that explicitly incorporates morbidity. This second approach, which is based on the notion that many diseases are interdependent, raises the possibility that the answer to the question posed at the beginning of this section might well be less than 15 percent. Because of interdependence there may be a tendency for the death rate from the other diseases to decline, and this tendency may offset the opposite effect of competing risks on that death rate.

A General Approach to the Modeling of Mortality Risks with Disease Interdependence

In this section we provide a more formal description of the approach set forth in the discussion associated with Figure 2–2. The objective is to derive a procedure for the specification of a model that will predict the mortality effects of specific health improvements while allowing for interdependence between diseases. This can be done in four logical stages as follows:

1. Specify a morbidity function for each disease (or group of diseases), showing for the population in question the determinants of the morbidity rate:

$$p_i = p_i(\mathbf{A_i}, p_j) \qquad i, j = 1, 2, \ldots, n \qquad (i \neq j) \qquad (2\text{–}1)$$

   where p_i is the fraction of the population (defined by age, sex, or other characteristics) who have disease i at some time during a defined time interval. There are n diseases. Each morbidity rate p_i is determined by a set of socioeconomic, environmental, and policy variables represented by the vector $\mathbf{A_i}$ and also by the prevalence of each other disease p_j. Degrees of interdependence are measured by the partial derivatives $\partial p_i/\partial p_j$. The impact of policy variables is measured by the partial derivatives $\partial p_i/\partial \mathbf{A_i}$.

2. Define all possible combinations of diseases and derive from the morbidity functions the fraction of the population having each combination:

$$c_k = c_k(p_i) \qquad (2\text{–}2)$$

   where $k = \bar{1}23 \ldots n$, $1\bar{2}3 \ldots n$, $12\bar{3} \ldots n$, for a total of $(2^n - 1)$ such terms; $(\bar{1}23 \ldots n)$ is read as "having all diseases except Disease 1" and where c_k is the fraction with disease-combination k. If there are n diseases, there will be $(2^n - 1)$ disease combinations. For example, in a two-disease system a person may have Disease 1 but not Disease 2, may have Disease 2 but not Disease 1, or may have both diseases, for a total of three possible disease combinations. Clearly the c_k are mutually exclusive (unlike the p_i), and the following relationship also holds true:

$$\sum_k c_k + c_w = 1 \qquad (2\text{–}3)$$

where c_w is the fraction of the population who remain well (or have diseases excluded from the analysis) throughout the entire interval. In addition the generated rates must be consistent with the elementary postulates of probability theory.[12]

3. For each disease combination, specify a fatality function, showing what determines the fatality rate among those with a given disease combination:

$$f_k = f_k(\mathbf{B_k}) \qquad (2\text{–}4)$$

where f_k is the fraction of those with disease combination k who die during the specified time interval, and $\mathbf{B_k}$ is a vector of socioeconomic, environmental, and policy variables. Specifying fatality functions in this way allows for the sort of phenomenon noted by Chiang in the quotation cited above: that a person who has cardiovascularrenal disease in combination with some other disease may have a probability of dying different from that of a person who has only that other disease.

4. Multiplying a fatality rate (f_k) by the corresponding disease-combination rate (c_k) then gives the fraction of the entire population who die from that particular disease combination during the interval in question (d_k):

$$d_k = f_k \cdot c_k \qquad (2\text{–}5)$$

And because the c_k's are mutually exclusive, the sum of the d_k's equals the general death rate D:[c]

$$D = \sum_k d_k \qquad (2\text{–}6)$$

[c] This derivation of D can be compared with that appearing in a series of health planning models developed by Correa (*Population, Health, Nutrition*, pp. 117–169), whose expression for D, using our notation, is as follows:

$$D = \sum_{i=1}^{n} (f_i \cdot p_i)$$

But since the morbidity rates p_i are not mutually exclusive, this formulation obviously overstates D.

The programming application of a model derived using this approach is consistent with the schema introduced in Figures 1–1, 2–1, and 2–2. An intervention designed to reduce mortality, such as mass vaccination against measles, will cause changes in the vectors $\mathbf{A_i}$ or $\mathbf{B_i}$. A simulation exercise with the model will therefore show the effects of the intervention on the general death rate D, with full allowance being made for both interdependence and competing risks. A heuristic advantage of the approach, it might be noted, is that public health interventions involving "prevention" affect $\mathbf{A_i}$, while those involving "treatment" affect $\mathbf{B_i}$.

Specification of a Morbidity-Mortality Model

Several steps must be taken in order to use the approach outlined above for the specification of a morbidity-mortality model in a given application. First, a form must be chosen for the functions generating the marginal morbidity rates (equation 2–1). Second, assumptions must be made and a procedure developed that will allow the transition between the marginal disease rates to the mutually exclusive joint disease rates (equation 2–2). Third, a form must be chosen for the fatality rate functions (equation 2–4).

The manner in which these steps are taken is arbitrary and will vary with the particular situation to be modeled. The steps outlined below form the basis for the initial computer simulation model we developed for the infant mortality project. The procedure to be used for the specification of the coefficients (see Chapter 5) is intended to be flexible enough to allow experiments with other equation forms. The optimization technique is intended to be sufficiently flexible to allow the use of alternative treatments of the probability constraints needed for the probability transition relationships.

Marginal Morbidity Rates. To derive a functional form for the marginal morbidity rates, we commence with the general form (equation 2–1), which we assume to be continuous and differentiable and note that changes in the rate of disease i are related to changes in other disease rates and to changes in policy variables by the differential equation:

$$dp_i = \sum_{j \neq i} \frac{\partial p_i}{\partial p_j} dp_j - \frac{\partial p_i}{\partial \mathbf{A_i}} d\mathbf{A_i} \tag{2–7}$$

Since the morbidity rates, p_i, are interpreted as probabilities, equations (2–1) and (2–7) must satisfy the following boundary conditions: if $p_i = 1$ or 0, then dp_i must equal zero for changes in p_j and $\mathbf{A_i}$. It can be demonstrated[13] that the algebraically simplest specification that can satisfy these conditions is the logit

$$p_i = \frac{1}{1 + \exp\left(-\gamma_i - \alpha_i \mathbf{A}_i - \sum_{j \neq i} \beta_{ij} p_j\right)} \qquad (2\text{–}8)$$

where $\beta_{ij} = \partial p_i / \partial p_j$ and α_i is a vector with the policy impact derivatives, $\partial p_i / \partial \mathbf{A}_j$ as elements. γ_i is a constant that is chosen after values for α_i, β_i, and $\mathbf{A}_i$ and initial values for p_i and p_j are given.

Transition from Marginal to Joint Disease Rates

Consistency. In general it is not possible to go from a marginal distribution to a joint distribution without assumptions regarding the kind and degree of relationships among the events whose distributions are being considered. For example, the simplest assumption one might make is that the events are independent; it then follows that the joint rates can simply be obtained as the product of the marginal rates. However, if there are interdependencies among events, as there are with the disease events we are considering, the generation of joint relationships quickly becomes more complicated. One of the problems is that the probabilities generated must be consistent with the elementary postulates of the calculus of probability.[d] Given a particular choice of functional form, the consistency requirement imposes relationships on the parameters of the probability functions. Consistency can be achieved by solving analytically for the required relationships between parameters, by specifying consistent functional forms, or by repeated testing of values generated by the model and the rejection of inconsistent solutions. When the model has more than two or three diseases, the analytical solution for consistent parameters or the derivation of consistent functional forms becomes intractable. For our initial simulation model, we have decided to use the second alternative—that is, to impose constraints (boundary values) on the probabilities generated, which will force the solutions produced in the optimization program to be consistent with the postulates of probability theory. Thus, resource allocation choices that produce probabilities outside the boundaries will be found to produce suboptimum solutions and successive allocations will be made until the generated probabilities are consistent with the probability constraints.

[d] The problem is analogous to one that occurs in the estimation of demand systems in economics. There the estimated system should be consistent with the elementary theorems of utility theory. In practice one of two procedures can be used: (1) a system of equations yielding consistent solutions is used for estimation; or (2) a less restrictive system of equations is used and the estimated parameters are tested for consistency.

Calculation of Joint Disease Rates. The generation of the joint disease rates is accomplished through their decomposition into components distinguished by the presence or lack of a causal influence between diseases. The problem has been simplified by assuming that there is no mutual causation, that is, the probability that i leads to j and j to i in a given individual over a given time period is zero. It is also assumed that joint causation is negligible, that is, the probability that i and j together cause k is zero. Finally the probability of more than three diseases is set to zero under the assumption that the loss in accuracy is negligible. An exposition of the derivation of the joint disease rates for a four-disease model is given in Appendix 2A. The derivation for a two-disease model is given in the next section.

A Two-Disease Model of Interdependence

We now specify an interdependence model with a view to providing a numerical illustration, choosing the simple case of only two diseases or disease groups. The numbering of the equations in this specific model follows that used in the general model above. It will be noted that the most complex part of the specific model lies in the derivation of the disease-combination rates c_k.

The morbidity rate for Disease 1 (p_1) is determined by the rate for Disease 2 (p_2) and by an index of other factors (a_{10}):

$$p_1 = \frac{1}{1 + e^{-(a_{10}+a_{12}p_2)}} \tag{2–1a}$$

And similarly for Disease 2:

$$p_2 = \frac{1}{1 + e^{-(a_{20}+a_{21}p_1)}} \tag{2–1b}$$

where a_{12} and a_{21} are indexes of interdependence. As we noted above, the particular functional form chosen for these equations (the logit form) has the property of constraining the morbidity rates to lie between zero and one.[e]

The disease-combination rates $c_{\bar{1}2}$ and $c_{1\bar{2}}$ are readily derived as follows:

$$c_{\bar{1}2} = p_2 - c_{12} \tag{2–2a}$$

$$c_{1\bar{2}} = p_1 - c_{12} \tag{2–2b}$$

where c_{12} is the fraction of the population having both diseases. If the two

[e] The inclusion of the simultaneous terms directly in the logit is used in this example only. In the larger model used in other chapters the terms enter linearly. The specification of the linear interaction terms in the larger model is discussed in detail in Chapter 3.

Table 2–1. Disease Combinations with Two Interdependent Diseases.

	Has Disease 1 caused by Disease 2	*Has Disease 1 not caused by Disease 2*	*Does not have Disease 1*	*Row Sum*
Has Disease 2 caused by Disease 1	0	$c_{1\to 2}$	0	$c_{1\to 2}$
Has Disease 2 not caused by Disease 1	$c_{2\to 1}$	$c_{(12)}$	$c_{2\bar{1}}$	$p_2 - c_{1\to 2}$
Does not have Disease 2	0	$c_{1\bar{2}}$	c_w	$1 - p_2$
Column sum	$c_{2\to 1}$	$p_1 - c_{2\to 1}$	$1 - p_1$	1

Note: Entries in the matrix represent the fraction of a population with the characteristics indicated.

diseases were independent, it would be reasonable to assume that this fraction was equal to the product of the two morbidity rates:

$$c_{12} = p_1 \cdot p_2 \tag{2–2c}$$

But with interdependence, equation (2–2c) is not valid. With interdependence, c_{12} must be measured by adding together (i) cases where Disease 1 causes Disease 2 ($c_{1\to 2}$), (ii) cases where Disease 2 causes Disease 1 ($c_{2\to 1}$), and (iii) cases where both diseases occur but without any causal link between them ($c_{(12)}$). The point is clarified in Table 2–1. Each disease may be caused by the other, not caused by the other, or not present at all. Considering both diseases, there are then nine categories into which the population may fall. Three of these are eliminated on logical grounds.[f] The remaining six are mutually exclusive.

By examination of Table 2–1 we therefore conclude that

$$c_{12} = c_{1\to 2} + c_{2\to 1} + c_{(12)} \tag{2–2d}$$

Separate expressions must now be obtained for the three components of c_{12}. The fraction of the population where Disease 1 causes Disease 2 can be measured as the *difference* between (i) the fraction actually having Disease 2 (p_2) and (ii) the fraction who would have Disease 2 if Disease 1 did not exist (that is, if $p_1 = 0$). Symbolically

[f]First, a person who "does not have Disease 1" cannot have during the same time interval "Disease 2 caused by Disease 1." (Lagged effects, as when Disease 1 occurring in one period causes Disease 2 to occur in the next, can be readily incorporated into a dynamic version of the model.) Second, a person who "does not have Disease 2" cannot have "Disease 1 caused by Disease 2." Third, cases of mutual causation are ruled out, where a person has "Disease 1 caused by Disease 2" as well as "Disease 2 caused by Disease 1." It is assumed that within the given time interval, one of the diseases will occur first and cannot therefore be caused by the other.

$$c_{1\rightarrow 2} = p_2 - \frac{1}{1 + e^{-a_{20}}} \qquad \text{(2–2e)}$$

Similarly

$$c_{2\rightarrow 1} = p_1 - \frac{1}{1 + e^{-a_{10}}} \qquad \text{(2–2e)}$$

The fraction of the population where both diseases exist without causal connection ($c_{(12)}$) can be reasonably estimated as the product of two independent frequencies: (i) the frequency of having Disease 1 not caused by Disease 2; and (ii) the frequency of having Disease 2 not caused by Disease 1. That is

$$c_{(12)} = (p_1 - c_{2\rightarrow 1}) \cdot (p_2 - c_{1\rightarrow 2}) \qquad \text{(2–2g)}$$

The three disease-combination rates $c_{\bar{1}2}$, $c_{1\bar{2}}$, and c_{12} having been determined, the next step is to specify the corresponding fatality rates $f_{\bar{1}2}$, $f_{1\bar{2}}$, and f_{12}. To simplify this version of the interdependence model, the fatality rates are assumed to be fixed.[g] We then have equations for the disease-combination–specific death rates $d_{\bar{1}2}$, $d_{1\bar{2}}$, and d_{12}:

$$d_{\bar{1}2} = f_{\bar{1}2} \cdot c_{\bar{1}2} \qquad \text{(2–5a)}$$

$$d_{1\bar{2}} = f_{1\bar{2}} \cdot f_{1\bar{2}} \qquad \text{(2–5b)}$$

$$d_{12} = f_{12} \cdot c_{12} \qquad \text{(2–5c)}$$

and for the general death rate D:

$$D = d_{\bar{1}2} + d_{1\bar{2}} + d_{12} \qquad \text{(2–6a)}$$

The operation of the model is illustrated with a numerical example in Table 2–2. It is imagined in column (B) that information is available on the morbidity rates p_1 and p_2, for example from a morbidity survey of households. Information also exists on the partial derivatives $\partial p_1/\partial p_2$ and $\partial p_2/\partial p_1$, which can be interpreted as the likelihood that one disease will lead to the other (within the given time interval). This information may be obtainable from analysis of individual medical histories. Given p_1, p_2, and the two derivatives, the a terms in the morbidity functions can be derived as well as the disease-combination rates (c_k).[h] With fatality rates (f_k) also supplied, the general death rate D can then be calculated.

g In the larger mortality model presented in Chapter 3, the fatality rates are generated as a linear function of the type of curative care.

h The calculation of the a terms involves using the following for the two derivatives:

$$\partial p_1/\partial p_2 = a_{12} e^{-(a_{10} + a_{12} p_2)} [1 + e^{-(a_{10} + a_{12} p_2)}]^{-2} \qquad \text{(2–7a)}$$

$$\partial p_2/\partial p_1 = a_{21} e^{-(a_{20} + a_{21} p_1)} [1 + e^{-(a_{20} + a_{21} p_1)}]^{-2} \qquad \text{(2–7b)}$$

Table 2–2. Hypothetical Effects of Disease Elimination on Mortality in a Two-Disease System with and without Interdependence.

		With Interdependence		*Without Interdependence*	
	Equation(s) from which derived (A)	*Both diseases present (B)*	*Disease 1 eliminated (C)*	*Both diseases present (D)*	*Disease 1 eliminated (E)*
1. p_1	2–1a	.1500*	0	.1500*	0
2. p_1	2–1b	.4000*	.3488	.4000*	.4000
3. $\partial p_1/\partial p_2$	2–7a	.1000*	0	0	0
4. $\partial p_2/\partial p_1$	2–7b	.3500*	—	0	0
5. a_{10}	2–1a, 2–7a	−2.0483	−∞*	−1.7346	−∞*
6. a_{12}	2–1a, 2–7a	.7843	.7843*	0*	0*
7. a_{20}	2–1b, 2–7b	−.6242	−.6242*	−.4055	−.4055*
8. a_{21}	2–1b, 2–7b	1.4583	1.4583*	0*	0*
9. $c_{1\to 2}$	2–2e	.0512	0	0	0
10. $c_{2\to 1}$	2–2f	.0358	0	0	0
11. $c_{(12)}$	2–2g	.0398	0	.0600	0
12. $c_{\bar{1}2}$	2–2a	.2667	.3488	.3400	.4000
13. $c_{1\bar{2}}$	2–2b	.0167	0	.0900	.4000
14. c_{12}	2–2d	.1333	0	.0600	0
15. f_{12}		.2500*	.2500*	.2500*	.2500*
16. $f_{\bar{1}2}$		.3000*	.3000*	.3000	.3000*
17. $f_{1\bar{2}}$		.4000*	.4000*	.4000*	.4000*
18. $d_{\bar{1}2}$	2–5a	.0667	.0872	.0850	.1000
19. $d_{1\bar{2}}$	2–5b	.0050	0	.0270	0
20. d_{12}	2–5c	.0533	0	.0240	0
21. D	2–6a	.1250	.0872	.1360	.1000

Note: Values marked with asterisks are assumed; remaining values are derived from the equation(s) indicated.

In column (C), the effects of eliminating Disease 1 are shown. To eliminate the disease, the value of a_{10} is changed to $-\infty$. The other a terms remain the same as in column (B), and the morbidity rate for the remaining disease is recalculated. The disease-combination rates are also affected and the general death rate falls by 30 percent.

Columns (D) and (E) show what happens if the two diseases are independent. The same model is used (except that zero values are assumed for the interdependence terms a_{12} and a_{21}), and the same initial values are assumed for the morbidity and fatality rates. The elimination of Disease 1 reduces the general death rate by 26 percent. As would be expected, this reduction is smaller than the result in an interdependent system.

Table 2–2 also suggests how to answer the question about death rates that was posed at the beginning of this chapter. It is evident that the answer depends on how cases with both diseases are handled in the statistics on causes of death. If deaths of persons with both Disease 1 and Disease 2 are officially attributed to Disease 1, then the elimination of Disease 1 will cause the general death rate to fall by an amount *less than* the official death rate for Disease 1, regardless of any interdependence. With this kind of record keeping, the death rate from Disease 1 is $(d_{1\bar{2}} + d_{12})$. The general death rate is always $(d_{\bar{1}2} + d_{1\bar{2}} + d_{12})$. Eliminating Disease 1 reduces $d_{1\bar{2}}$ and d_{12} to zero but necessarily raises $d_{\bar{1}2}$ (because of competing risks). Hence the fall in the general death rate will be less than $(d_{1\bar{2}} + d_{12})$, or the official death rate from Disease 1.

If, however, deaths of persons with both diseases are officially attributed to Disease 2, the elimination of Disease 1 could lower the general death rate by *more* than the official death rate for Disease 1. Table 2–2 shows this happening both with and without interdependence. When the death rate for Disease 1 is defined as $d_{1\bar{2}}$, the elimination of that disease will lower the general death rate $(d_{\bar{1}2} + d_{1\bar{2}} + d_{12})$ by more than the death rate for Disease 1 if the rise in $d_{\bar{1}2}$ (due to competing risks) is less than d_{12}.

SUMMARY

An approach to modeling the mortality process has been developed. By separating mortality into morbidity and fatality components the approach provides for a distinction between preventive and curative interventions. Using a two-disease example the approach was contrasted with the theory of competing risks. It was found that, unlike the existing theory of competing risks, the procedure devised here allows for disease interdependence in the calculation of an estimate of the mortality effects of disease elimination (or reduction). By specifying the structure of the model in terms of marginal disease rates, rather than mutually exclusive joint disease rates, the number of parameters needed for specification of a given model is significantly reduced.

The approach devised here is sufficiently general to be applied in a variety of contexts. In Chapter 3 the approach is used to specify a model of child mortality covering the first sixty months of life.

NOTES

1. See Martin Feldstein, M. A. Piot, and T. K. Sundaresan, *Resource Allocation Model for Public Health Planning: A Case Study of Tuberculosis Control*, World Health Organization, Geneva, 1973.
2. For instance, see Hector Correa, *Population, Health, Nutrition and Development* (Lexington, Mass.: Lexington Books, 1975), Chapter 5.
3. *Ibid.*, p. 134.

4. P. S. Heller and W. D. Drake, *Malnutrition, Child Morbidity, and the Family Decision Process*, University of Michigan, Center for Research on Economic Development, Discussion Paper No. 58 (Ann Arbor, Mich., 1976).
5. A. Rashmi, D. K. Guha, and P. C. Khanduja, "Postmeasles Pulmonary Complications in Children," *Indian Pediatrics* 8 (1971): 834–838.
6. P. Newman, *Malaria Eradication and Population Growth* (Ann Arbor, Mich.: Bureau of Public Health Economics, 1965).
7. C. L. Chiang, "On the Probability of Death from Specific Causes in the Presence of Competing Risks," *Fourth Berkeley Symp. IV* (1961): 169–180; and C. L. Chiang, "Competing Risks and Conditional Probabilities," *Biometrics* 26 (1970): 767–776.
8. A. W. Kimball, "Models for the Estimation of Competing Risks from Grouped Data," *Biometrics* 25 (1969): 329–337.
9. C. L. Chiang, "On the Probability of Death from Specific Causes," p. 172.
10. Kimball, "Models for Estimation of Competing Risks," pp. 332–333.
11. Chiang, "Competing Risks," p. 775.
12. See Norman C. Dalkey, "An Elementary Cross Impact Model," *Technological Forecasting and Social Change* 3 (1972), reprinted in Harold A. Linstone and Murray Turoff, eds., *The Delphi Method* (Reading, Mass.: Addison-Wesley, 1975), pp. 327–337.
13. For a demonstration and the development of a cross-impact analysis based on a logit specification of behavioral probability functions, see Murray Turoff, "An Alternative Approach to Cross Impact Analysis," *Technological Forecasting and Social Change* 3 (1972), reprinted in Linstone and Turoff, eds., *The Delphi Method*, pp. 338–368.

Appendix 2A

Algebraic Summary of the Morbidity–Mortality Model

This appendix presents a summary of the general morbidity-mortality model described heuristically in the text. The objective in the design of the model is to allow the calculation of a set of mortality rates for mutually exclusive morbidity categories that includes all possible combinations of diseases. There are four distinct segments to the system. The first involves the specification of a set of marginal probabilities as functions of interventions as well as other variables. This segment can be referred to as that of the structural (or causal) morbidity equations. The second segment is a set of algebraic relationships that allows the calculation of the probabilities of being in the mutually exclusive joint disease states. The third segment involves the specification of fatality probabilities for each of the mutually exclusive categories. This segment can be called the structural fatality equations. Finally, the fourth segment uses the fatality rates and joint morbidity rates to calculate the mortality rate.

I. Structural Morbidity Equations

In the current project the model is developed for four diseases. The extention to n diseases is straightforward although tedious. We specify the following marginal morbidity functions for Diseases 1, 2, 3, and 4:

$$p_1 = p_1(\mathbf{A}_1, p_2, p_3, p_4) \qquad (2A\text{–}1)$$

$$\vdots$$

$$p_4 = p_4(\mathbf{A}_1, p_2, p_3, p_4) \qquad (2A\text{–}4)$$

II. Calculation of Mutually Exclusive Joint Disease Rates

a. *Preliminary definitions:*

i. p_{ij} is the probability of having i and j jointly.

ii. p_{ijk} is the probability of having i, j, and k jointly.

iii. $\tilde{p}_{ij}$ is the probability that i occurs caused by j, that is

$$\tilde{p}_{ij} = p_i(\mathbf{A}_i, p_j \cdots p_l) - p_i(\mathbf{A}_i, p_k \cdots p_l)\Big|_{p_j=0}$$

iv. Similarly

$$\tilde{p}_{ijk} = p_i(\mathbf{A}_i, p_j \cdots p_l) - p_i(\mathbf{A}_i, p_l)\Big|_{p_j, p_k=0}$$

v. p^*_{ij} is the probability that i occurs and is not caused by j, that is,

$$p^*_{ij} = p_i - \tilde{p}_{ij}$$

vi. Similarly

$$p^*_{ijk} = p_i - \tilde{p}_{ijk}$$

b. *Preliminary assumption:*

It is assumed that intersection probabilities of order higher than three are zero, that is, $p_{1234} = 0$

c. *Preliminary calculation—two-disease intersections:*

There are two kinds of cases where two diseases can occursimultaneously:

i. no causal links between diseases

ii. the two diseases are linked causally (either i causes j, or j causes i, or both). Thus the two-disease intersection for i and j can be written using the notation introduced above as

$$p_{ij} = \tilde{p}_{ji} + \tilde{p}_{ij} - \tilde{p}_{ij} \cdot \tilde{p}_{ji} + p^*_{ij}p^*_{ji}$$

d. *Preliminary calculation—three-disease intersections:*

There are eight kinds of cases where the three diseases can occur simultaneously:

	Diagrammatically
i. no causal links between the 3 diseases	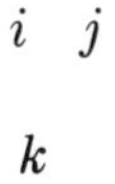 i j k
ii. i and j are causally linked (either i causes j, or j causes i, or both), but k is not causally linked with either i or j	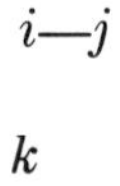 i—j k
iii. i and k linked, j independent	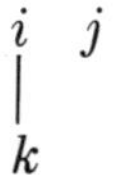 i j | k
iv. j and k linked, i independent	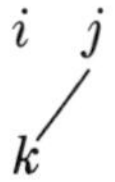 i j / k
v. i and j linked, also i and k, but not j and k	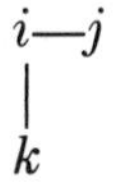 i—j | k
vi. i and j linked, also j and k, but not i and k	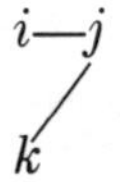 i—j / k
vii. i and k linked, also j and k, but not i and j	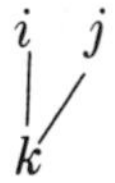 i j | / k
viii. i and j linked, also i and k, also j and k	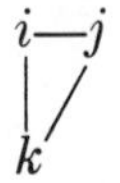 i—j | / k

The eight groups being mutually exclusive, p_{ijk} is the sum of all eight. Keeping the eight groups in order, and defining

$$x_{ij} = [\tilde{p}_{ij} + \tilde{p}_{ji} - \tilde{p}_{ij} \cdot \tilde{p}_{ji}]$$

the three-disease intersection can be written as the sum of eight terms.

$$\begin{aligned} p_{ijk} = p^*_{ijk} \cdot p^*_{jik} \cdot p^*_{kij} & \\ + x_{ij}p^*_{kij} & \\ + x_{ik}p^*_{jik} & \\ + x_{jk}p^*_{ijk} & \\ + x_{ik}x_{jk}(1 - x_{ij}) & \\ + x_{ij}x_{jk}(1 - x_{ik}) & \\ + x_{ij}x_{ik}(1 - x_{jk}) & \\ + x_{ij}x_{ik}x_{jk} & \end{aligned}$$

e. Given the preliminary calculations above, the rates for the mutually exclusive disease states can be derived as follows:

   i. $c_{1\overline{234}} = p_1 - p_{12} - p_{13} - p_{14} + p_{123} + p_{124} + p_{134} - p_{1234}$
      $c_{2\overline{134}} = p_2 - p_{12} - p_{23} - p_{24} + p_{123} + p_{124} + p_{234} - p_{1234}$
      ⋮
      and so on for $c_{3\overline{124}}$ and $c_{4\overline{123}}$.

   ii. $c_{12\overline{34}} = p_{12} - p_{123} - p_{124} + p_{1234}$
      ⋮
      and so on for $c_{13\overline{24}}$, $c_{14\overline{23}}$, $c_{23\overline{14}}$, $c_{24\overline{13}}$, and $c_{34\overline{12}}$.

   iii. $c_{123\overline{4}} = p_{123} - p_{1234}$
      ⋮
      and so on for $c_{124\overline{3}}$, $c_{134\overline{2}}$, and $c_{234\overline{1}}$.

   iv. the states defined above + p_{1234} + p_{well} will sum to one. (We have assumed that p_{1234} is negligible.)

III. Structural Fatality Functions

Fatality functions are specified for each of the joint disease states.

$$d_1 = d_1(\mathbf{B}_1)$$
$$\vdots$$
$$d_K = d_{15}(\mathbf{B_K})$$

where K is the total number of disease states ($K = 2^n - 1 = 15$).

IV. The Mortality Rate.

The mortality rate can be derived as the sum of the mortality rates for the individual joint disease states.

$$D = \sum_{k=1}^{K} d_k c_k$$

Chapter 3

The Child Mortality Model

INTRODUCTION

This chapter describes the full child mortality model that will be used in the optimization program. Diseases, disease relationships, and potential interventions that are appropriate in the context of given age groups for the childhood period in a peripheral urban community in a developing country are identified and then the model is specified using the general approach discussed in Chapter 2. The model is designed to compare the effectiveness of alternative interventions in the reduction of excess child mortality. Before commencing with a discussion of diseases and interventions, we define excess mortality and discuss the breakdown of the first five years of life into appropriate age groups.

Obligatory Versus Excess Mortality

In order to limit the range of the analysis to morbidity and mortality rates that are reasonable given the state of technology and physiological reality, bounds are placed on the probability functions. The effect of the bounds will be to restrict the optimization search to plausible reductions in morbidity and mortality rates given the available technology and practicable interventions in a developing country.

The whole concept of mortality under the age of five may be analyzed under two main categories: (1) those deaths that might be avoided by the broader application of known measures; and (2) those deaths that could only be prevented by the discovery and application of new methods. For the practical purpose of the specification of the optimization model, it is possible to use developed or industrialized countries' mortality rates as "obligatory losses" or deaths that can only be prevented by the discovery and application of new medical and public health technology in developed countries. Mortality rates above this fundamental minimum could be considered "excess losses," potentially reducible by extending services and changing the environment in developing countries.

For developed countries, the mortality rates during childhood (1–14 years) are lower than during any other period over the life span. Decreases in the risk of mortality continue throughout the childhood period after the first few weeks of life. The death rate in the preschool age group (1–4 years) has always been a small fraction of the infant mortality rate; in the United States in recent years it has been less than 5 percent of the rate under one year of age. In fact, in the United States 96.4 percent of all deaths under the age of five occurred in the first year of life. Over 40 percent of the deaths during the first year occur in the first day, 65 percent in the first week, and 70 percent in the first month. These deaths, at least from the point of view of our model, can be attributed to unavoidable physiological causes and most of the decrease in mortality rates in developed countries over the last twenty years can be accounted for by the significant changes after the first week of life. Observation of mortality rates in developed areas thus gives a kernel of unavoidable mortality that is fairly large in the first few weeks of life but quickly tapers off to very low values for the remainder of the childhood period.

If the rates and mortality structure attained at the present time by developed countries are defined as the portion of deaths that are "obligatory," anything above could be considered preventable. A plausible upper bound can be obtained through the use of data for a region and time where there was little or no preventive or curative activity and environmental conditions were extremely poor. The reduction in mortality below this upper bound can then be attributed to health intervention activities and changing environmental and socioeconomic conditions.

In the child mortality model, the upper and lower bounds on morbidity and fatality rates will be specified algebraically by an appropriate choice of α_U and α_L in functions of modified logit form,

$$p = \alpha_L + \frac{\alpha_U}{1 + e^{-Z}}$$

This function is illustrated in Figure 3–1. As Z, which is a function of inter-

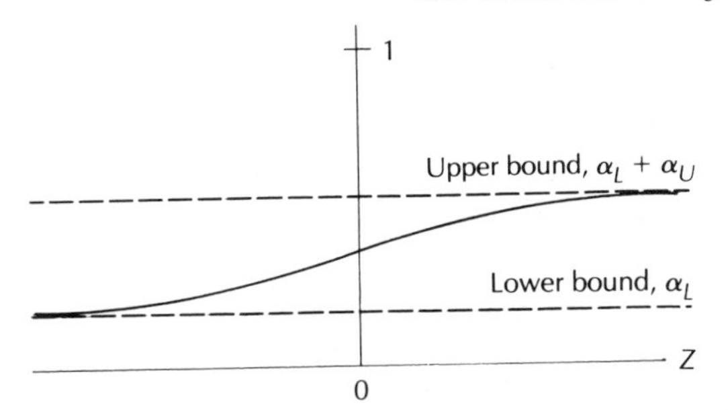

Figure 3–1. Example of a constrained morbidity function (logit form).

vention activities and sociological variables, becomes very large and negative, p approaches the lower limit, α_L. Conversely, as Z becomes very large and positive, p approaches the upper limit, $\alpha_L + \alpha_U$. With α_U and $\alpha_L + \alpha_U$ set, respectively, to values from countries with the most and least favorable conditions for infant survival, the values for the morbidity and fatality rates generated by the model can be restricted to a plausible range.

Choice of Age Groups

Because morbidity risks and responses to interventions change with the physical development of a child, we have divided the overall period under analysis, the first sixty months of life, into three separate age groups. The division chosen is the neonatal period (the first month of life); the infant period (1–12 months of life); and the toddler period (12–60 months). These three periods are set apart from each other by large differences in mortality associated with distinct physiological characteristics in the development of the child. The first month of life is marked by a high risk of death from low birth weight and what we have called "obligatory causes." The period from one to twelve months is characterized by relative immobility of the child, breast feeding, and transferred maternal immunity for some childhood diseases. In contrast, the period from twelve to sixty months is characterized by increased contact with the environment and susceptibility to the immunizable diseases of childhood. For the thirteen countries of the PAHO mortality study,[1] the average neonatal mortality rate was 39.7 per 1000 live born (24.2 to 49.4). For the infant period (twenty-ninth day to eleven months) the rate was 39.8 of 1000 live born (14.6 to 83.9). The rate for children one to four years was 6.2 (1.5 to 26.2).

The entire model therefore actually consists of three submodels covering three different age groups in the span between birth and five years of age. Individual age groups are linked in that the survivors of younger age groups become the demographic basis for intervention coverage and morbidity rates in the older age group.

DISEASE CATEGORIES

The selection of diseases used in the model is guided by three criteria. First, the objective of the model is to include a minimum number of morbidity states for simplicity but to account for at least 75 percent of childhood mortality. Second, diseases that have well-known and obvious interventions that might be thought cost effective prior to a formal analysis are included. The first two criteria might conflict, for instance, tetanus and childhood inoculable diseases may account for less than 10 to 15 percent of childhood mortality in some ares. (Although in other areas, such as parts of India, their importance is indisputable.[2]) But the existence of vaccination toxins of known efficacy dictated the inclusion of these disease categories in the model.

The final criterion is a comparison of mortality rates by cause and age of death in developed and less-developed regions or a comparison of mortality rates for developed countries over time to identify disease categories that show the most potential for reduction. This was the basis for the monu-

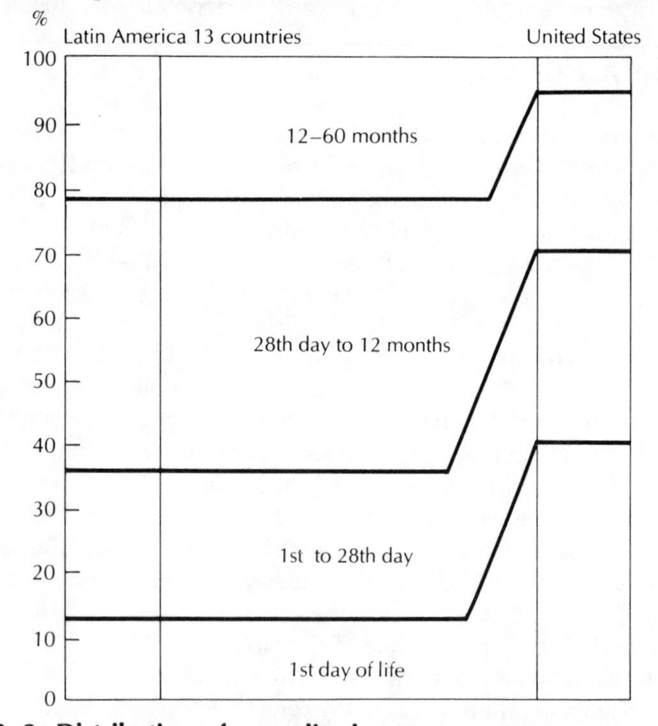

Figure 3–2. Distribution of mortality by age groups as percent of child deaths in Latin America and the United States. *Source:* Ruth Puffer and Carlos Serrano, eds., *Patterns of Mortality in Childhood,* Pan American Health Organization, Scientific Publication No. 262, Washington, D.C., 1973, pp. 371–428.

mental study by Puffer and Serrano[3] and is perhaps the most important criterion since it identifies a very few diseases with a great potential for improvement. The age-specific rates of death in developing countries grossly follow the same pattern as those in developed countries with a high proportion of deaths occurring at very early stages of life. The magnitude, however, is different. Small differences between less-developed and more-developed countries are found in the rates for the first day of life (maximum twofold). The difference increases steadily however to rates 10 to 15 times higher at ages two to four years.

A comparison of mortality rates for Cali, Colombia, and California indicates that, for the neonatal group, there are marked differences in the rate of low-birth-weight deliveries and in the mortality rates for categories where low birth weight is either a contributing or underlying cause. This apparent interactive relationship is especially important with respect to neonatal infection. Together these two categories explain a substantial proportion of neonatal deaths. To these two categories is added neonatal tetanus, which has obvious associated interventions and which is almost nonexistent in the United States, but is a significant cause of mortality among newborn children in developing areas. Finally, because there are major differences in the way the delivery is handled in developed and developing countries, birth trauma is added as a fourth category.

The major cause of mortality among infants in the one-to-twelve month group in developing countries is gastrointestinal infection. An examination of changes in childhood mortality rates in Europe and the United States shows that the primary reason for the great reduction in rates over the last thirty to fifty years has been the near elimination of diarrhea as a cause of infant death. A second reason for the dramatic reduction in mortality rates is the decrease in the rate of childhood mortality from respiratory infections. Both respiratory infections and diarrhea have potential synergistic relationships with malnutrition. In particular, the interrelationship between diarrhea and malnutrition has been the subject of extensive research. Further, evidence supports the observation that malnutrition is an important associated cause of death and significantly increases the fatality rates for other diseases when present. To these three diseases is added the category of immunizable disease for which only whooping cough is significant during the first twelve months.

The disease categories explaining the differential between developed and developing country childhood mortality rates remain essentially unchanged for the one-to-four year age group. The immunizable disease category, however, becomes more significant with measles and polio developing as potential causes of mortality as neonatal immunities are lost and increased exposure to the environment occurs. In addition the interaction between immunizable diseases and malnutrition becomes sufficiently substantial to warrant being included in the model.

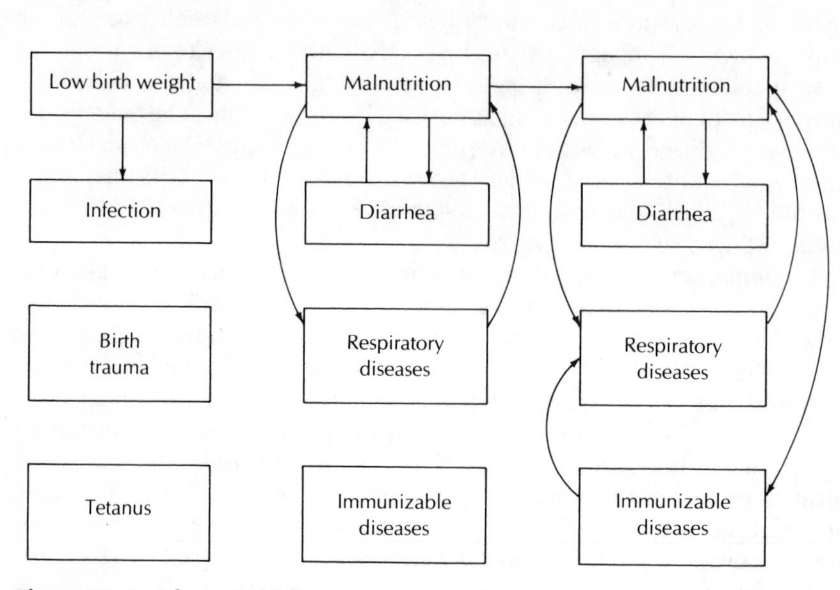

Figure 3–3. The morbidity segment of the child mortality model (showing interdisease causal flows).

The diseases included in the analysis account for over 80 percent of childhood mortality in less-developed countries. The selection of diseases thus holds out the potential for a significant reduction of mortality both because the diseases account for a large part of mortality in developing areas and because known interventions have already brought about a significant decline in their incidence in developed countries.

The diseases and their interrelationships are summarized in Figure 3–3. The arrows connecting the diseases indicate the direction of a potential causal flow that will be included in the model in the form of a nonzero interaction coefficient (for the disease to which the arrow runs) in the marginal probability function (see equation (2–7) in Chapter 2). Only the most significant disease interactions are included. The importance of the disease interrelationships is that they allow for indirect effects of interventions that, if not included, might cause the effectiveness of particular interventions to be underestimated. For instance, malnutrition is not a significant direct cause of mortality; it is, however, an important contributor to higher morbidity rates for other diseases. In addition, the fatality rates for respiratory and immunizable diseases are higher for malnourished children. Thus a nutritional supplement may be potentially cost effective in mortality reduction even though direct deaths through starvation or nutritional deficiencies are small in number.

The next few pages are concerned with a definition of the disease categories used in the infant mortality model, especially with an explanation of the degree of aggregation used, and with an outline of the types of interventions to be considered. The interventions are described in more detail in a following section. The concern here is with a brief description of the potential mode of impact of interventions on the diseases. Since the importance of these diseases and their interrelationships is well known and previously documented the discussion is cursory.

Low Birth Weight

For the purposes of this study, low birth weight is defined as a weight of 2500 grams or less immediately after delivery. This definition encompasses two subcategories of births, each of which may arise for different reasons. The most important of these categories in developing countries and the category to which we devote most of our attention is low birth weight attributable to a deficiency in nutrients reaching the fetus. This can occur because of a malfunctioning of the placenta and/or a deficiency of nutrient intake by the mother before or during pregnancy. The second subcategory is children born prematurely who are of lower weight because of a shorter fetal development period. This group, which may be the result of nonnutritional physiological problems of either the mother or fetus, does not behave as malnourished and may be less responsive to interventions.

The interventions considered for the reduction of morbidity in the low-birth-weight category are aimed at increasing the quantity and quality of nutrients reaching the fetus and at decreasing the opportunity for a malfunction of the pregnancy. Classified by target group, the interventions are aimed at (1) women not presently pregnant but capable of conception; (2) pregnant women; and (3) women known to have a high risk of giving birth to a low-birth-weight child (because of previous birth histories or present nutritional and physiological status).

Interventions for nonpregnant women within the reproductive age bracket involve health education and promotion, good health care access, and access to good nutrition. The general categories of activities that might be accomplished are: avoiding pregnancies at the extremes of the reproductive age bracket (less than eighteen or over thirty-five years of age), avoiding pregnancies within two years of a previous pregnancy, providing treatment for malnourished female adults within the reproductive age bracket, and providing education on hygiene and nutrition to women within the reproductive age bracket.

Interventions for pregnant women are aimed at early detection and appropriate remedial treatment of factors known to be associated with low birth weight. Thus the intervention activities include: early detection of pregnancy; early detection of anemia, urinary tract infection, venereal disease, toxemia, hypertension and diabetes; encouragement of cooperation in prenatal control; and nutritional supplements during pregnancy.

Birth Trauma

Birth trauma is referred to as the pathological process occurring because of or as a consequence of delivery. It may be produced by misfunctioning of the birth process, misfunctioning of the birth canal, mishandling of the delivery by the mother or person attending (helping) the delivery, or malformations in the development of the fetus that produce interference with the proper transit through the birth canal. Prior to delivery, interventions to reduce birth trauma include the early detection and treatment of diabetes, toxemia, and hypertension. With early detection of pelvic malformations, birth canal obstruction, or other indications of a high-risk delivery, adequate facilities for instrumental or surgical delivery might be provided.

Neonatal Infections

Two broad categories of neonatal infection are aggregated under this heading. The first is superficial or localized infections such as pyodermitis, conjunctivitis, and moniliasis. The second is systemic infections such as respiratory tract infections, neonatal diarrhea, and sepsis. The infections can also be classified by transmission agent or source, that is, those transmitted from the mother through the placenta to the fetus, those produced by direct contact of the child with the birth canal, and those acquired through environmental contact after birth. Generally, the interventions to reduce morbidity through infection are intended to act through a reduction of the possibility of transmission by controlling infection in the mother and by controlling the condition of the neonatal environment.

Interventions on pregnant women include detection and treatment of venereal disese, viral diseases, and infections of the birth canal, and control of the mother's environment to reduce the opportunity for maternal infection. Interventions on the child and neonatal environment include control of the delivery environment, profilaxis of the eyes and cord at birth, and appropriate care of caput or scalp hemorrhages. Finally, breast feeding and counsel of the mother on breast and feeding hygiene is a potentially important activity intended to control the neonatal environment.

Tetanus

Tetanus neonatorium is usually produced by improper handling of the umbilical cord. The activities to reduce tetanus are immunization of the mother during pregnancy and appropriate care of the umbilical cord during and after delivery.

With regard to curative interventions, neonatal tetanus is of sufficient severity that combination disease states with tetanus are aggregated to a single mutually exclusive disease state. The assumption is that the presence of tetanus will be an overriding factor in the determination of treatment and the calculation of fatality rates for all disease states where tetanus is present. Outpatient care is assumed to have little usefulness and the only care we are considering in this study is intensive inpatient care with appropriate facilities.

Malnutrition

Malnutrition is a deficit of major nutrients with respect to standard requirements that will produce retarded growth and development in children of a reference population. We are using the Gomez[4] standards as the criterion and include malnutrition of degrees II and above in this morbidity category. Malnutrition can occur with a decrease in the intake and absorption of nutrients or an increase in the requirements for nutrients or both simultaneously. Thus, a change in the volume of nutrients metabolized may not only occur as a consequence of a food deficiency, but may also occur because of metabolic changes produced by infection or the lack of absorption of the nutrients due to gastrointestinal pathology.

Interventions that affect the level of malnutrition directly are concerned with increasing the quality and quantity of nutrient intake. These include: nutritional education for the mother, especially concerning complementary foods, and the encouragement of breast feeding; improving lactation of the mother up to the weaning age; and supplementary weaning foods. Other interventions that affect malnutrition indirectly through a reduction in gastrointestinal infection are considered under diarrhea.

Although malnutrition is an uncommon cause of death when not associated with other diseases, it frequently severely increases the fatality rate of other morbidity conditions when it is found in association with them. The choice of curative care is dependent on the associated disease. Outpatient treatment of all grades of malnutrition consists of activities similar to those designed to reduce morbidity.

Diarrhea

In this study diarrhea is defined as "a disturbance of intestinal motility and absorption which once and by whatever means produced, may become self perpetuating as a disease through the production of dehydration and profound cellular disturbances, which in turn favor the continuing passage of liquid stools."[5] Diarrhea, as defined, is a symptom and can be a result of any of a great number of enteropathogen or physiological causes.

The morbidity interventions to be considered are primarily intended to act on the reduction of enteropathogen transmission by controlling the child's environment and reducing the opportunity for indirect fecal contact. Thus the interventions should be directed to provide potable water, a clean environment, maternal personal hygiene, a clean bottle, and maintenance of breast feeding as long as possible.

Three processes produce death when a child has diarrhea: dehydration, dissemination of infection (sepsis), and starvation. Both inpatient and outpatient care are intended to attack the three processes by providing early and adequate replacement of fluids, adequate treatment of infections by antibiotics where necessary, and nonlactose foods for early refeeding.[a] The essential difference between outpatient and inpatient treatment is the opportunity for observation and control, and the use of rehydration facilities in the health center.

Respiratory Diseases

At the level of aggregation used in this study, the heading "Respiratory Diseases" refers to acute lower respiratory tract infections with the addition of acute bronchitis, pneumonia, and tuberculosis. Specifically excluded are mild upper respiratory problems and immunizable respiratory diseases of childhood. The morbidity interventions are intended to reduce transmission through maternal education and control of the environment. Maternal education and participation in a well-baby clinic may also reduce the incidence in this category by providing adequate treatment of upper respiratory infections.

Immunizable Diseases

This category includes whooping cough and measles (eleventh and twelfth month only) in the infant age groups and diphtheria, whooping cough, tetanus, measles, and polio in the toddler age group. Morbidity interventions include inoculations and environmental control.

ACTIVITIES FOR THE REDUCTION OF CHILD MORTALITY

The interventions to be considered in this study are defined in terms of activities. Each activity consists of the execution of procedures or techniques involved in the control of various morbidity or fatality categories. The distinction between activities and interventions lies in the

[a] The important effect of treatment for diarrhea may not be so much on fatality from diarrhea as upon the diarrhea-malnutrition link.

usage of the health services. An activity is defined in terms of the number of units of a given service that are *available* but not necessarily used. An intervention is the effective proportional coverage of a given target group by an activity actually used. For example, the available scale of a nutritional program may be sufficient to cover 80 percent of all children but if participation is not sufficiently promoted only half of the available service will actually be used. In this case, although the per capita coverage of the program is potentially 0.8, the value of the intervention is only 0.4.

A further distinction between interventions and activities is made with regard to services for prenatal care. In this case, the timing of the use of the services is important and available prenatal care activities are split between interventions depending on whether the activity is delivered with early detection of pregnancy in the first trimester or without early detection in the second or third trimesters. The proportion of prenatal care in each intervention category is determined by a prenatal care usage function.

Two activities, examinations for all women and examinations for pregnant women, do not enter directly in the determination of any intervention. These two activities affect the level of several interventions indirectly through a series of restrictions that require examinations and tests before certain activities can be carried out. An example of an intervention of this type is an examination of potential mothers and tests for various diseases including iron deficiency and then treatment for iron-deficient women. The intervention thus involves two activities (1) examination and tests; and (2) treatment of iron deficiency.

Activities are, therefore, the variables that are scaled by the program in the allocation of resources. Interventions are related to the activities through comparisons with usage demand and a number of special relationships involved in the actual delivery of services. The interventions then become the arguments in the morbidity and fatality functions determining the level of mortality.

Table 3–1 presents a list of the activities as well as the socioeconomic variables assumed to have an impact on the morbidity, fatality, and usage functions for each age group and disease included in the model. A number code used to identify the activities is included in the left-hand column. The intervention comprising the test and treatment of women of childbearing age for anemia thus involves activity 2 and activity 5. A more detailed description of the activities follows the table.

Table 3–1. Inventory of Activities to Reduce Child Mortality and Socioeconomic Variables Affecting Mortality.

Task Code[a]	
	A. *Age 0–1 month*
	I. Health Post-Health Center
	1. Prenatal Care—pregnant women only
3	a. Examination and tests, then if needed:
7	i. Treatment of venereal disease, anemia, urinary tract infection, toxemia, hypertension, and diabetes
8	ii. Nutritional supplement for low-birth-weight-risk mothers only
15	iii. Delivery of low-birth-weight- and birth-trauma-risk mothers in health center
9	b. Tetanus immunization of mothers
10	c. Hygienic education and nutritional counseling in health center
11	d. Nutritional program for all pregnant women (could be delivered without health post-health center)
	2. Health care for all women of childbearing age
2	a. Examination and tests, then if needed:
	i. Treatment of venereal disease and urinary tract infections
6	ii. Treatment of anemia for iron-deficient women only
5	b. Anemia program for all women (delivered by promotora)
	II. Delivery
12	1. In health center, by midwife or auxiliary nurse, doctor on call
	2. In home
13	a. by midwife trained in eye and cord profilaxis
14	b. unattended, eye and cord profilaxis given later by promotora
	III. Postnatal Care (impact on both morbidity and mortality)
16	a. Outpatient care for low birth weight and infections
17	b. Inpatient care—specific treatments for low birth weight, birth trauma, infections, and tetanus
	IV. Water
	1. Adequate quantity and quality
18	a. In home
19	b. Within a short walk (100 meters)
	V. Sanitation
	1. Excreta disposal
20	a. In-house hygienic toilet facilities connected to sewage system or septic tank
21	b. Latrines, outside, not connected to sewage system
	VI. Program Usage
	1. Effect on use of prenatal care, nutrition program, postnatal care, and breast feeding of:
	a. educational level of household
	b. household income

[a] The code is used to identify the tasks in algebraic formulations of the model and in computer programming. The numbering corresponds to that used in the structural equation tables at the end of this chapter. Only the first occurrence of the task is numbered.

Table 3–1. *(Continued)*

Task Code[a]	
22	c. mass media (specific messages)
	d. promotora
1	VII. Promotora (three visits per year)
	Services provided by promotora
	1. Hygienic and nutritional education
	2. Early detection of pregnancy and referral
	3. Detection of infections and malnutrition of women and referral (if. I.2., above, is used)
	VIII. Socioeconomic Variables and Health Status
	a. income
	b. education
	c. income/family size
	d. family size
	e. sq. meters of housing/family size
	f. age of mother
	g. birth interval
	B. Age 1–12 months
	I. Promotora (three visits for 1–12 month age group)
	Services provided by promotora related to 1–12 month age group.
	1. To detect malnourished child, respiratory infections, severe diarrhea, and then make referral
	2. To encourage breast feeding
	3. To provide nutritional and hygienic education and evaluation
	4. To encourage use of health center services for check up or shots (if programs are used)
	II. Health Post-Health Center
23	1. DPT, polio, and measles immunization alternative #1
24	2. Well-baby clinic—routine check-up (first visit to doctor, last three to auxiliary nurse) and referral at 3, 4, 6, and 12 months, nutritional education
25	3. Nutritional supplement for child (could be promoted without health center)
26	4. Nutritional supplement for breast-feeding mother
27	5. Outpatient care for 1–12 month age group as appropriate for diarrhea, respiratory, or inoculable diseases
28	6. Inpatient care for 1–12 month age group as appropriate for diarrhea, respiratory, or inoculable diseases
	III. Water
	1. Adequate quantity and quality
	a. In home
	b. Within a short walk (100 meters)
	IV. Sanitation
	1. Excreta disposal
	a. In-house hygienic toilet facilities
	b. Latrines
	V. Program Usage
	1. Effect on use of preventative care, nutrition program, breast feeding, and curative care of:

Table 3–1. *(Continued)*

Task Code[a]	
	a. educational level of mother
	b. household income
	c. mass media
	d. promotora
	VIII. Socioeconomic Variables and Health Status
	a. income
	b. education
	c. income/family size
	d. family size
	e. sq. meters of housing/family size
	C. Age 12–60 months
	I. Promotora (three visits per year)
	1. To detect malnourished child, respiratory infections, severe diarrhea, and then make referral
	2. To provide nutritional and hygienic education
	3. To encourage use of health center services for check up or shots (if programs are used)
	II. Health Center
	1. Continuation of DPT, polio, measles immunization
	2. Well-baby clinic—routine check up by auxiliary nurse and referral at 24, 36, and 48 months, nutritional education
30	3. Nutritional supplement for child
31	4. Outpatient care for 12–60 month age group as appropriate for diarrhea, respiratory, or inoculable diseases
32	5. Inpatient care in health center for 12–60 month age group as appropriate for diarrhea, respiratory, or inoculable diseases.
	III. Water
	1. Adequate quantity and quality
	a. In home
	b. Within short walk (100 meters)
	IV. Sanitation
	1. Excreta disposal
	a. In-house hygienic toilet facilities
	b. Latrines
	V. Program Usage
	1. Effect on use of preventative care, nutritional program and curative care of:
	a. educational level of mother
	b. household income
	c. mass media
	d. promotora
	VIII. Socioeconomic Variables and Health Status
	a. income
	b. education
	c. income/family size
	d. family size
	e. sq. meters of housing/family size

DESCRIPTION OF INTERVENTION ACTIVITIES[b]

Activity 1. Health Promoter (PROMOTER). The promotora, in the program we are considering, is a nonprofessional health worker who is given specific messages and assigned limited services to deliver in visits to the household every four months. Promotoras are usually women between eighteen and twenty-five years old with at least seven years of primary education who receive approximately two to three months of training. They live in the areas in which they work and are generally accepted as inside members of the community. The mother is their usual contact in the household.

In the child mortality model the actions of the promotora are differentiated according to whether or not they promote the usage of health services or provide a direct service themselves. This distinction is preserved in the survey questions regarding the impact of the promotora.

The most important functions of the promotora that have a potential direct effect on morbidity are educational. Specifically the promotora provides education about personal and child hygiene and the proper use of water and sanitary services. Nutritional advice concerning the choice and preparation of foods is also given. The promotora also teaches the mother to look for signs of morbidity and how to care for mild illness. Other, noneducational service tasks are considered under appropriate intervention headings.

The primary function of the promotora is to promote the use of health services. In this function she identifies, for the mother (or prospective mother), existing health services in the community and encourages the use of the services where appropriate. She also attempts to detect pregnant women, within the first trimester, for referral to a health center for a prenatal exam. The promotora may also be used as part of a program to encourage breast feeding.

Activity 2. Examination and Tests for Women of Childbearing Age (AWEXAM). This activity consists of an annual examination by paramedical personnel (a registered nurse or equivalent training) in a health center with a medical doctor available for consultation. The objective is to identify fertile women with conditions that might affect the quality of a pregnancy and fetal development. Of specific concern, because related activities are to be considered, are tests for the existence of venereal disease, other genito-urinary tract infections, and anemia.

[b] The headings are followed by short labels to be used to identify activities in the tables in the remainder of this chapter.

Activity 3. Examination and Clinical Tests for Pregnant Women (PWEXAM). This activity consists of an examination, in a health center or health post, of women with suspected pregnancy. The objective of the examination is to confirm pregnancy and screen women for medical problems that would complicate the pregnancy or detract from optimal fetal growth. Specifically, the tests are concerned with venereal disease, genito-urinary tract infections, hypertension, diabetes, toxemia, anemia, and malnutrition. The examination is made by a medical doctor or by a paramedic under the supervision of a doctor.

In the survey questions regarding the effectiveness of the examination and related treatment, a distinction is made between an exam and treatment carried out in the first trimester of pregnancy (and, thus, possibly in conjunction with a program for early detection of pregnancy) and an exam and treatment carried out later in the pregnancy. An exam and treatment sequence for prenatal care consists of three health center visits during pregnancy.

Activity 4. Treatment of Venereal Disease and Urinary Tract Infection (AWTXINF). This activity is the outpatient treatment, through a health center, of venereal disease and urinary tract infection in fertile women of reproductive age. The treatment consists of an appropriate prescription of antibiotic drugs and the encouragement of cooperation in carrying through with the treatment and continued observation.

Activity 5. Anemia Program for All Women (AWTXANE). This activity consists of the fortification of food with iron in a dose sufficient to prevent anemia.

Activity 6. Treatment of Anemia for Iron-Deficient Women Only (AFEDEFTX). This treatment consists of the prescription of an iron supplement for anemic women and encouragement of participation in the program. The difference between activities 5 and 6 is the target group. In activity 5 all women, whether presently anemic or not, receive an iron supplement. The supplement and encouragement of participation can be delivered either through the health center or by a promotora. In activity 6 the target group is presently anemic women. In addition to the supplement and encouragement of participation, activity 6 includes continued observation and measurement.

Activity 7. Treatment of Morbidity Conditions in Pregnant Women (PWTXINF). This activity consists of outpatient treatment of venereal disease, anemia, genito-urinary tract infection, toxemia, diabetes, hypertension, and anemia. The treatments, consisting of drugs and counsel as appropriate, are administered through a health center.

Activity 8. Nutritional Supplement for Low-Birth-Weight-Risk Mothers (PWNUTLBW). This activity consists of the introduction of a protein-calorie and iron supplement equal to the average deficit identified in the community under analysis. The supplement is given only to households having pregnant women with a high risk of giving birth to a low-birth-weight infant.

Activity 9. Tetanus Immunization of Pregnant Women (PWTETIMM). The tetanus immunization is delivered by a promotora on one of her three visits per year or in the health center. The immunization is given before the eighth month of pregnancy.

Activity 10. Hygienic Education and Nutritional Counseling in a Health Center (PWHCED). In this activity pregnant women are counseled by a paramedic, registered nurse, or doctor on the importance of good nutrition and hygienic habits during pregnancy. The content of the messages is standard medical practice and the counseling occurs as part of a visit to a health center for examination. Education and counsel given by the promotora are not considered as part of this intervention.

Activity 11. Nutritional Program for All Pregnant Women (PWNUT). In this activity, pregnant women are given a protein-calorie and iron supplement equal to the average deficit for women of childbearing age in the community. This activity differs from activity 8 in that the supplement is given to all pregnant women without regard to their nutritional status.

Activity 12. Delivery in a Health Center (DELIN). Delivery is assisted in a health center by a trained midwife or registered nurse. The health center employs a medical doctor, has an ambulance, and is equipped for a normal delivery. The delivery personnel are trained to recognize abnormalities in the development of the delivery that call for referral to a regional hospital.

Activity 13. Delivery at Home Attended by Midwife (DELMW). The midwife attending the home delivery in this intervention task is trained to recognize signs of an abnormal delivery for referral to a health center. The midwife is recognized as a member of the community and has received training in treatment for asepsia and eye and cord profilaxis.

Activity 14. Promotora Visit after an Unattended Home Delivery (DELPROM). Within forty-eight hours of an unattended delivery, a promotora visits the home and gives eye and cord profilaxis and advice on the adequate care of the umbilical cord. The promotora also attempts to recognize neonatal problems for referral to a health center.

Activity 15. Delivery of High-Risk Births in a Health Center (DELINLBW). This activity takes place in a health center and consists of an examination, screening, and delivery of mothers with a high risk of low birth weight or a high risk of birth trauma.

Activity 16. Outpatient Neonatal Care (1OUTP). This activity consists of the current accepted treatment as needed for low birth weight and neonatal infections. The child is not hospitalized; the care is delivered through a health center with a physician available for counsel.

Activity 17. Inpatient Neonatal Care (1INP). This activity consists of the current accepted inpatient treatment and care as needed for low birth weight, birth trauma, infection, and tetanus. The care is given in a health center with back up services available as required at a regional hospital.

Activity 18. In-Home Piped Water (H2OHOME). This activity consists of the provision of potable water in sufficient quantity for drinking, cooking, and household sanitation. The water is piped to the household and available through at least one spigot.

Activity 19. Public Fountain (H2OWALK). An adequate quality and quantity of water is available at a public fountain within 100 meters of the household. Note that in both this activity and activity 18 the quality of the water refers to the water at the tap and not necessarily as finally used. The quality of water usage (that is, the quality of handling and storage of water) is considered elsewhere.

Activity 20. In-House Toilet Facilities (TOILET). This activity consists of the provision of hygienic (flyproof) toilet facilities connected to a sewage system or septic tank.

Activity 21. Out-House Toilet Facilities (LATRINE). This activity consists of the provision of latrines, not connected to a septic tank or central sewage system, for each household. A cover for the latrine is provided, however, the latrine itself is not flyproof.

Activity 22. Mass Media (MMEDIA). In this activity, specific messages are delivered through advertising on the radio, on billboards, or in newspapers. The messages being considered are intended to affect the usage of health services and do not have a direct effect on morbidity.

Activity 23. DPT, Polio, and Measles Immunization (IMMDPTPM). The sequence of shots would be delivered at appropriate intervals by either a health promotor in a home visit or at the health center during visits to a well-baby clinic. The mode of delivery is assumed to affect usage levels and not the effectiveness of the shots.

Activity 24. Well-Baby Clinic, Infants (2WBC). This activity is carried out in the health center and consists of a routine checkup by a physician or registered nurse at three months followed by health center visits at four, six, and twelve months for routine examinations by an auxiliary nurse or paramedic. Nutritional and hygienic advice is given. Mothers are encouraged to use health services and referrals are made for treatment as needed.

Activity 25 and 30. Nutritional Supplement for Infants, Nutritional Supplement for Toddlers (2NUTCH and 3NUTCH). These activities consist in the provision of a protein-calorie supplement sufficient to close the nutritional gap for the average child in the community. It is assumed that the programs are designed in such a manner that the target group actually receives the supplement.

Activity 26. Nutritional Supplement for Breast-Feeding Mothers (2NUTBF). This consists of the protein-calorie supplement needed to close the gap between the community average and the standard requirements for breast-feeding women. The supplement is administered to breast-feeding mothers for six months.

Activities 27 and 31. Outpatient Care for Infants, Toddlers (2OUTP and 3OUTP). These activities consist of the provision of appropriate outpatient care for diarrhea, respiratory diseases, and inoculable diseases in the infant and toddler age groups. The care consists of an examination, tests, prescription of medicine, and advice. The care is given by trained medical personnel in a health center.

Activities 28 and 32. Inpatient Care for Infants, Toddlers (2INP and 3INP). These activities consist of the provision of inpatient care for diarrhea, respiratory illness, or inoculable diseases. The care is given in a health center or regional hospital as appropriate.

Activity 29. Well-Baby Clinic, Toddlers (3WBC). This activity consists of a routine checkup and nutritional counsel by an auxiliary nurse at twenty-seven, thirty-six, and forty-eight months.

STRUCTURAL EQUATIONS

There are three types of structural equations in the model. They generate the rates for intervention usage, marginal disease incidence, and fatality. By referring to Figure 2–1 and recalling the associated discussion in Chapter 2, the role of the three types of equations can be reviewed. As the arrows indicate, the usage rates (or, alternatively, participation rates), u_l, are calculated as a function of socioeconomic variables and intervention activities;

$$u_l = u_l(\mathbf{C}_l) \qquad l = 1 \ldots L \tag{3–1}$$

where $\mathbf{C}_l$ is a vector of appropriate socioeconomic variables and activities made up of the tasks described on the preceding pages; L is the total numbers of usage functions calculated. The usage rates are then compared with the available level of intervention programs per capita, x_i, and the minimum is selected to represent the level of interventions, I_i, used in the calculation of morbidity and fatality rates; that is,

$$I_i = \min \begin{Bmatrix} u_l \\ x_i \end{Bmatrix}$$

In actuality, the extent of program participation would be somewhat different for each intervention activity, since participation will vary with the perceived utility of each program as compared with the perceived costs. However, to keep the number of usage equations manageable, we have collected interventions into nine groups that might reasonably be expected to have similar participation characteristics and have specified individual usage functions for each group. The nine usage equations are:

1. Usage of prenatal care by all women,
2. Usage of prenatal care by pregnant women,

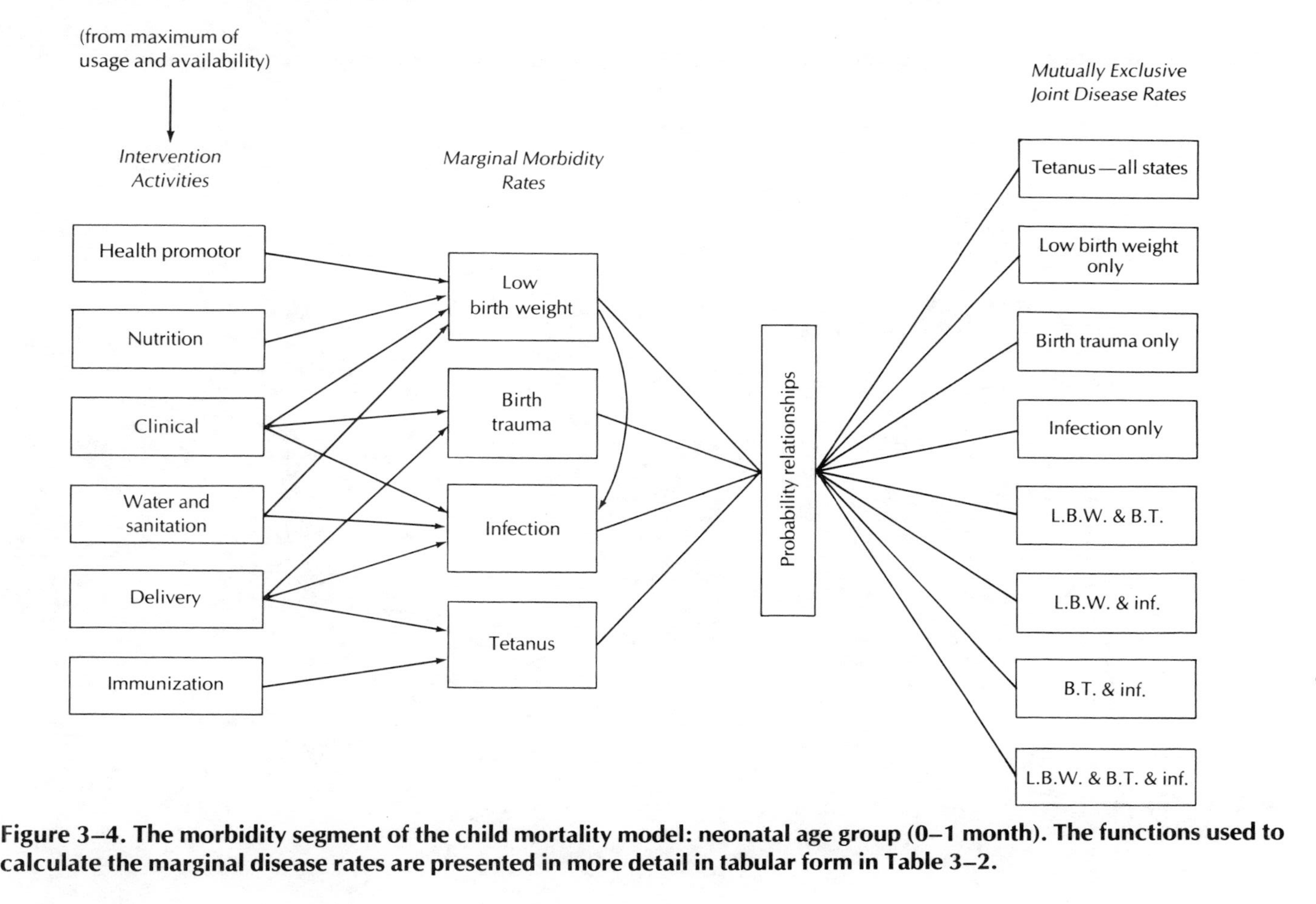

Figure 3–4. The morbidity segment of the child mortality model: neonatal age group (0–1 month). The functions used to calculate the marginal disease rates are presented in more detail in tabular form in Table 3–2.

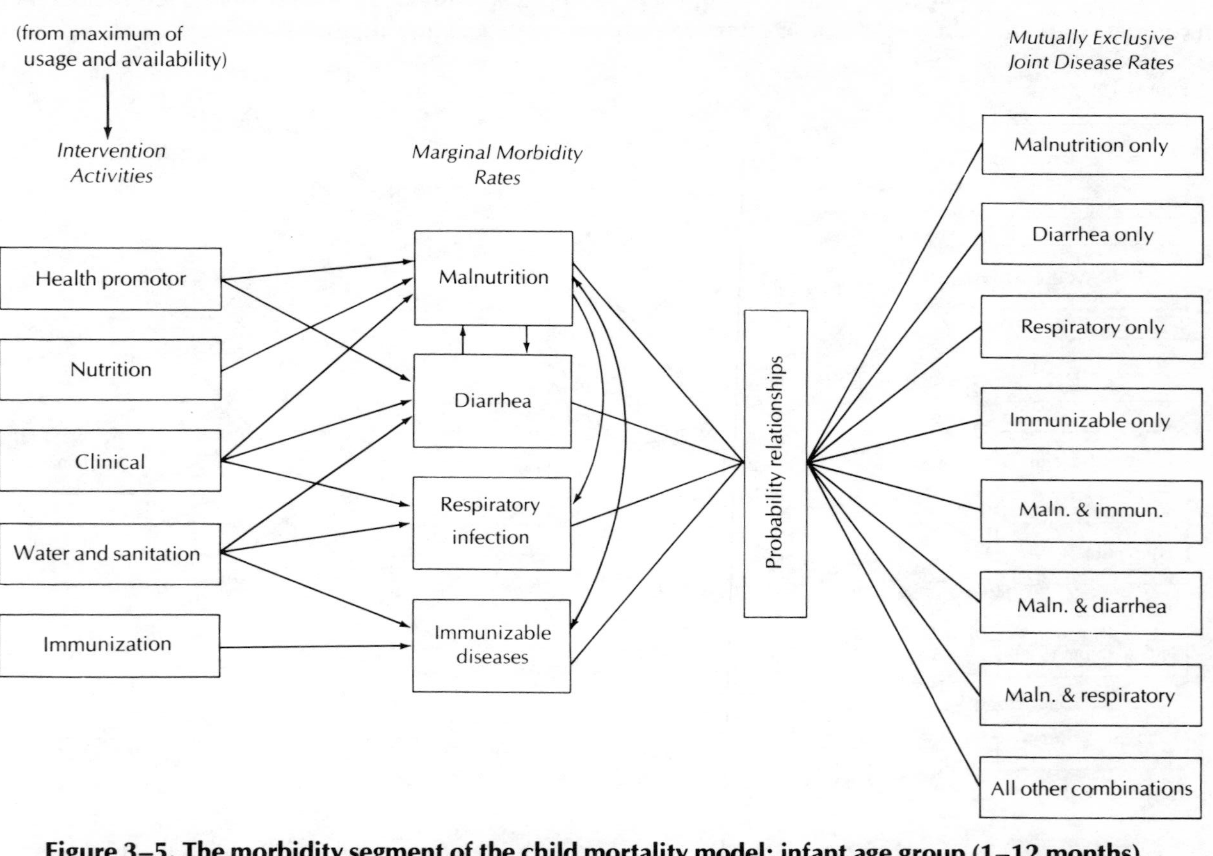

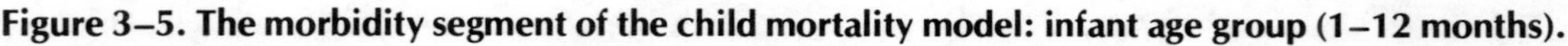

Figure 3–5. The morbidity segment of the child mortality model: infant age group (1–12 months).

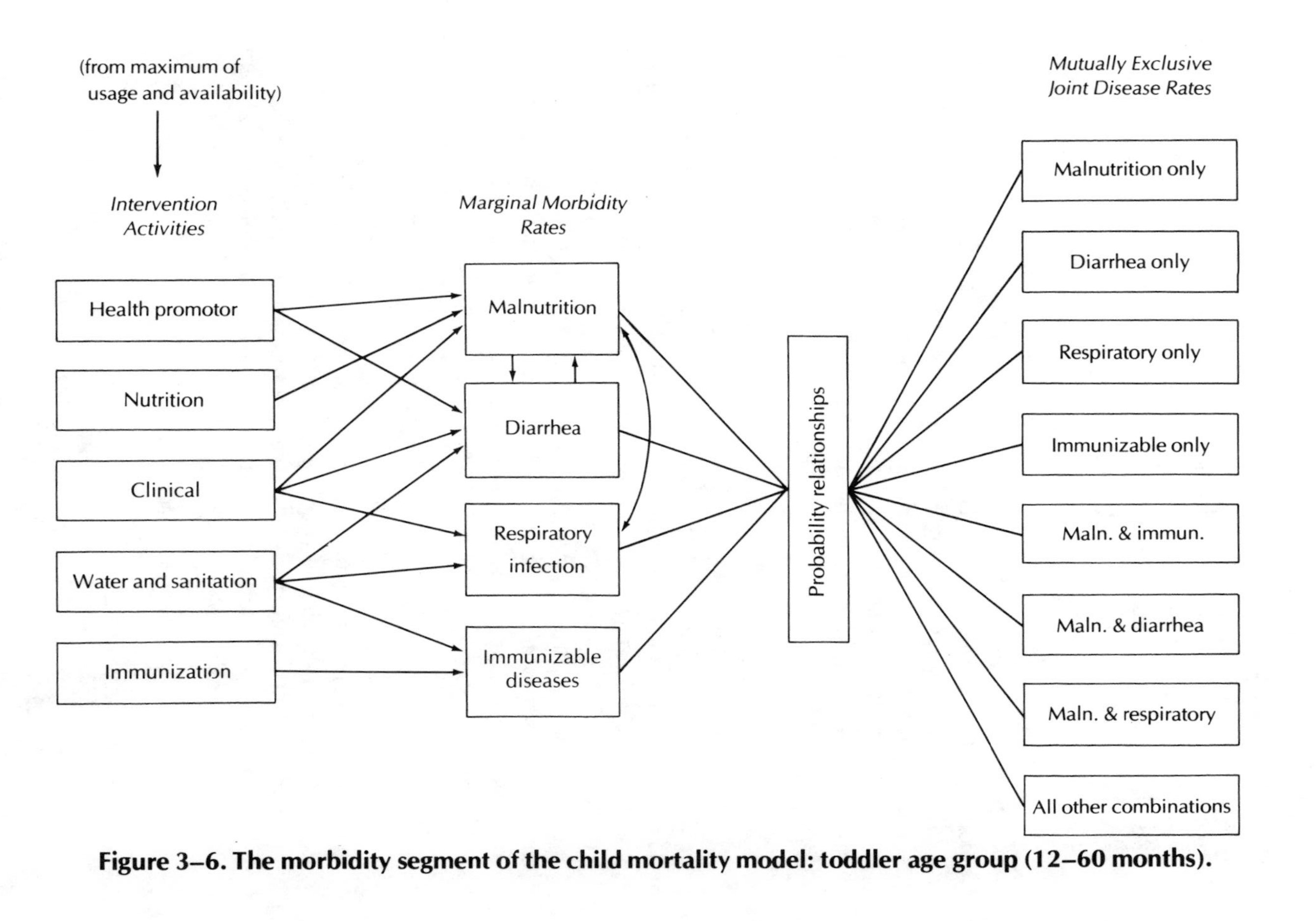

Figure 3–6. The morbidity segment of the child mortality model: toddler age group (12–60 months).

3. Usage of curative care,
4. Usage of breast feeding,
5. Proportion of prenatal care commenced in first trimester,
6. Usage of preventive care in the infant group,
7. Usage of curative care in the infant group,
8. Usage of preventive care in the toddler group, and
9. Usage of curative care in the toddler group.

The availability of each activity is compared with the applicable usage rate in deriving the minimum to be used as the effective level of the intervention in calculating the morbidity and fatality rates.[c] Thus, for example, the available capacity for prenatal obstetric examinations is compared with usage category 2 to determine the minimum representing the effective level of the obstetric examination intervention.

Given the effective level of the interventions, the age-specific morbidity rates can be calculated from the morbidity rate functions (see equation (2–1) in Chapter 2),

$$p_i = p_i(\mathbf{A}_\mathbf{i}, p_j) \qquad i, j = 1 \ldots n \quad i \neq j \tag{3–2}$$

The flows involved in these calculations are illustrated in Figures 3–4, 3–5, and 3–6. The boxes on the left represent the effective level of interventions derived from the procedure described in the previous paragraph. The interventions determine the marginal morbidity rates as shown by the arrows. In addition, the interactions among diseases are shown by the arrows drawn between various pairs of disease. Moving to the right the probability relationships (see equation (2–2) and Appendix 2A),

$$c_k = c_k(p_i) \qquad k = 1 \ldots K \tag{3–3}$$

are used to derive the mutually exclusive disease rates. Finally, if the derived rates are consistent with the constraints representing the primary postulates of probability theory (see the discussion in Chapter 2), the fatality rates are calculated using the fatality rate functions (see equation (2–4) in Chapter 2),

$$f_k = f_k(\mathbf{B}_\mathbf{k}) \qquad k = 1 \ldots K \tag{3–4}$$

and the mortality rate is obtained,

$$D = \sum_k f_k c_k \tag{3–5}$$

[a] With the exception of usage category 5. This category is used to partition prenatal care into early and late interventions.

The functional form chosen for the morbidity functions is a modified logit and the structural equations can be written as

$$p_{ia} = a_{ia} \left(\frac{\alpha_{iU}}{1 + e^{-Z_{ia}}} + \alpha_{iL} \right) + \\ + \sum_{j=1}^{n} b_{ija} p_{ja} + c_{ia} p_{i,a-1} \quad \begin{array}{l} i = 1 \ldots 4 \text{ (diseases)} \\ a = 1 \ldots 3 \text{ (age groups)} \end{array}$$

where $p_{i,a-1}$ represents the morbidity rate in the previous group, and Z_{ia} is a linear function of the various socioeconomic and intervention variables. The malnutrition equations for the last two age groups are the only morbidity functions given a lagged specification; thus c_{ia} is assumed to be equal to zero for all morbidity functions except p_{12}, p_{13}. The morbidity interaction terms, $b_{ija} p_{ja}$, are included linearly, instead of nonlinearly as in the example in Chapter 2, in order to simplify the solution of the simultaneous equations in the computer program.[d] In general, the choice of functional form is arbitrary as there is no precedent for this type of model. We have chosen the logit form as appropriately reflecting the behavior of many biological processes and to demonstrate the feasibility of using a nonlinear morbidity model for cost-effectiveness analysis. As experience with this type of model increases, other nonlinear forms may be found that provide a more accurate approximation of the processes involved; or, conversely, it may be found that linear functions are sufficient approximations of reality over the range of morbidity rates involved in specific problems. An algebraic derivation and interpretation of the functional form of the morbidity equations is given in Appendix 3A.

The functional form employed for the usage equations is the logit,

$$u_l = \frac{1}{1 + e^{-U_l}} \qquad l = 1 \ldots 9$$

where the U are linear functions of the socioeconomic and intervention variables. Again the choice of functional form was arbitrary and was made because of the convenient algebraic characteristics of the logit and because of the function's asymptotic properties.

The fatality rates are calculated as the weighted average of the fatality rates, f_{kah}, for each type of case. The weights, w_h, are the proportion of cases treated by each type of care. In the model specified here there are

[d] Nonlinear interaction terms are feasible, although costly in terms of computer time needed to obtain repeated solutions of the simultaneous morbidity functions.

three care possibilities—no care, outpatient, inpatient—and the fatality functions can be written,

$$f_{ka} = \sum_{h=1}^{3} w_h f_{kah} \qquad \begin{aligned} k &= 1 \ldots K \text{ (disease categories)} \\ a &= 1 \ldots 3 \text{ (age groups)} \\ h &= \text{type of care} \end{aligned}$$

The complete set of functions is summarized in Table 3–2. The functions are separated by age group and within age group by usage, morbidity, and fatality categories. To the right of the activities column, the functions are identified by dependent variable, u_1, P_2 and so on. (The age subscripts are omitted in the table.) The first column on the left names the independent variable; the second column gives the identifying subscript for the variables, and the third column identifies activities involved in the intervention activities.

To the right of the third column, a mark in the intersection between a row and a column indicates that the intervention activity or variable identified by the row is to be included as a variable in the equation identified by the column. There are two types of marks:

1. ✔ indicates simply that the variable is to be included.
2. U_l indicates that the minimum of U_l or x_i is to be used.

As an example of the use of the table, we write the equation for the usage of prenatal care by all women. This is found in the fourth column on the first page of the table for the neonatal age group. Noting that there are ✔s in the rows for promotora, mass media, household income, and education we write (omitting subscripts for the age group)

$$u_1 = \frac{1}{1 + e^{-U_1}}$$

with $$U_1 = \gamma_{1,0} + \gamma_{1,1} I_1 + \gamma_{1,24} I_{24} + \gamma_{1,41} S_1 + \gamma_{1,42} S_2$$

and where the γ are the elements of the C vector noted previously and are constants giving the impact of the various variables on U_1. The first subscripts on the coefficients identify the equation and the second subscripts identify the variable. The numbering of the coefficients on the socioeconomic variables is 40 plus the subscript of the variable; thus the coefficient on household income (socioeconomic variable number 1) is 41 (= 40 + 1).

As a second example, consider the morbidity function for respiratory disease in the toddler age group. Following the table we write (again omitting subscripts for the age group)

$$p_3 = \frac{\alpha_{3U}}{1 + e^{-Z_3}} + \alpha_{3L}$$

with

$$Z_3 = \alpha_{3,0} + \alpha_{3,22}U_4I_{22} + \alpha_{3,23}U_4I_{23} + \alpha_{3,34}I_{34} + \alpha_{3,44}S_4 + \beta_{3,1}P_1 + \beta_{3,4}P_4$$

where I_{34} is the minimum of X_{29} or U_8. Finally, as a third example, the fatality equation for the disease state "diarrhea only" in the infant age group is

$$f_2 = \delta_{2,0}(1 - I_{32} - I_{33}) + \delta_{2,32}I_{32} + \delta_{2,33}I_{33}$$

where I_{32} and I_{33} are the minimums of X_{27} and U_7, and X_{28} and U_7, respectively.

SUMMARY

This chapter has given a description of the simulation model that will be used to calculate the value of the objective in the optimization program. The model consists of four disease categories for each of three age groups. The age-specific disease rates are defined as a set of functions of thirty-seven health intervention activities and six socioeconomic variables. Figures 3–4, 3–5, and 3–6 summarize the relationships between the interventions and disease rates. Usage rates are generated as functions of health promotion interventions and socioeconomic variables. Table 3–2 defines the usage, morbidity, and fatality functions that comprise the structural equations of the model. Chapter 5 is concerned with the specification of the coefficients of the equations defined in Table 3–2.

NOTES

1. Ruth Puffer and Carlos Serrano, eds., *Patterns of Mortality in Childhood*, Pan American Health Organization, Scientific Publication No. 262, Washington, D.C., 1973.
2. See, for instance, G. B. Simmons, C. Smucker, B. D. Misra, and P. Majumdar, "Patterns and Causes of Infant Mortality in Rural Uttar Pradesh," *Journal of Tropical Pediatrics and Child Health* (October, 1978): pp. 207–216.
3. Puffer and Serrano, *Patterns of Mortality*.
4. F. Gomez, R. G. Galvan, J. Craviato and S. Frenk, "Malnutrition in Infancy and Childhood with Special Reference to Kwashiorkor," in S. Levine, ed., *Advances in Pediatrics*, Vol. 5 (New York: Year Book Publishers, 1955), p. 131.
5. World Health Organization Expert Committee, "Enterric Infections," WHO Technical Report Service, 1964, no. 288, p. 1.

Table 3–2. Structural Equations.

			Neonatal Age Group Usage Functions				
Activity or Variable	*Inter-vention Subscript Notation*	*Activities Involved (See Inventory of Activities)*	*Usage of Prenatal Care by All Women*	*Usage of Prenatal Care by Pregnant Women*	*Usage of Curative Care*	*Usage of Breast Feeding*	*Early Prenatal Care*
Intervention Activities	I_i	X_i	U_1	U_2	U_3	U_4	U_5
Promotora	1	1	✓	✓	✓	✓	✓
Exam & del. of high risk preg.	10	15			✓		
Delivery in health center	16	12			✓		
in home by midwife	17	13			✓		
in home w/ promotora later	18	14			✓		
Mass media	24	22	✓	✓	✓	✓	✓
Socioeconomic variables	S_i						
Household income	1		✓	✓	✓	✓	✓
Education	2		✓	✓	✓	✓	✓

Table 3–2. *(Continued)*

			Neonatal Age Group Morbidity Functions			
Activity or Variable	*Intervention Subscript Notation*	*Activities Involved*	*Low Birth Weight*	*Infection*	*Birth Trauma*	*Tetanus*
Intervention Activities	I_i	X_i	P_1	P_2	P_3	P_4
Promotora	1	1	✓	✓		
All women:						
exam and treat infection	2	2 + 4	U_1	U_1		
exam and treat anemia	3	2 + 6	U_1			
anemia program	4	5	U_1			
Pregnant women:						
exam and treat infection, etc.	5	3 + 7	U_2'	U_2'	U_2'	
exam and treat l.b.w. risk—nutrition	6	3 + 8	U_2'			
exam and del. of high risk pregnancies	7	3 + 15		U_2	U_2	U_2
tetanus immunization	7	9				U_2'
counsel in health center	8	10	U_2'	U_2'		U_2'
nutritional supplement—all preg.	9	11	U_2'			
Delivery						
in health center	16	12		U_2	U_2	U_2
at home by midwife	17	13		U_2	U_2	U_2

Note: $U_2' = U_2(1 - U_5)$

Table 3–2. *(Continued)*

Activity or Variable	Intervention Subscript Notation	Activities Involved	*Neonatal Age Group Morbidity Functions* Low Birth Weight	Infection	Birth Trauma	Tetanus
Intervention Activities	I_i	X_i	P_1	P_2	P_3	P_4
Delivery at home with promotora later	18	14		U_2		U_2
Breast feeding	19	U_4		✓		
Water: in home	20	18	✓	✓		
in public fountain	21	19	✓	✓		
Sanitation: in house toilet	22	20	✓	✓		
latrine	23	21	✓	✓		
Early detection of pregnancy:						
exam and treat for infection	11	3 + 7	U_2''	U_2''	U_2''	
nutritional supp. for l.b.w. risks	12	3 + 8	U_2''			
tetanus immunization	13	9				U_2''
counsel in health center	14	10	U_2''	U_2''		U_2''
nutritional program all pregnancies	15	11	U_2''			

Note: $U_2'' = U_2 U_5$.

Table 3–2. *(Continued)*

Activity or Variable	Intervention Subscript Notation	Activities Involved	Neonatal Age Group Morbidity Functions: Low Birth Weight	Infection	Birth Trauma	Tetanus
Socioeconomic Variables	S_i		P_1	P_2	P_3	P_4
Household income	1					
Education	2		✓	✓		
Household income per capita	3		✓	✓		
Number of rooms per capita	4			✓		
Age of mother: <18 years	5		✓		✓	
>35 years						
Birth interval < 2 years	6		✓		✓	
Simultaneous Variables	P_i					
Low birth weight	1			✓		

Activity or Variable	Intervention Subscript Notation	Activities Involved	Neonatal Age Group Fatality Functions: Tetanus, All States	Low Birth Weight Only	Birth Trauma Only	Infection Only	L.B.W. + B.T.	L.B.W. + Inf.	B.T. + Inf.	L.B.W. + B.T. + Inf.
Intervention Activities	I_i	X_i	f_1	f_2	f_3	f_4	f_5	f_6	f_7	f_8
Outpatient Care	25	16		U_3		U_3	U_3	U_3	U_3	U_3
Inpatient Care	26	17	U_3	U_3	U_3	U_3	U_3	U_3	U_3	U_3

Table 3–2. *(Continued)*

Infant Age Group Usage Functions				
Activity or Variable	*Subscript Notation*	*Activities Involved*	*Usage of Preventive Care, Infant Group*	*Usage of Curative Care, Infant Group*
Intervention Activities	I_i	X_i	U_6	U_7
Promotora	1	1	✓	✓
Mass media	24	22	✓	✓
Well-baby clinic, alt. #1	28	24		✓
Socioeconomic Variables	S_i			
Household income	1		✓	✓
Education	2		✓	✓

Infant Age Group Morbidity Functions						
Activity or Variable	*Subscript Notation*	*Activities Involved*	*Malnutrition*	*Diarrhea*	*Respiratory*	*Inoculable*
Intervention Variables	I_i	X_i	P_1	P_2	P_3	P_4
Promotora	1	1	✓	✓		
Water: in home	20	18		✓		
public fountain	21	19		✓		
Sanitation: in house toilet	22	20		✓	✓	
latrines	23	21		✓	✓	
Immunization: DPT, Polio, Measles	27	23				✓
Well-baby clinic	28	24	U_6	U_6	U_6	
Nutritional supp., child	29	25	U_6			
Nutritional supp., breast-feeding mother	30	26	U_4			
Breast feeding	31	U_4	✓	✓	✓	✓

Table 3–2. *(Continued)*

			Infant Age Group Morbidity Functions			
Activity or Variable	*Subscript Notation*	*Activities Involved*	*Malnutrition*	*Diarrhea*	*Respiratory*	*Inoculable*
Socioeconomic Variables	S_i		P_1	P_2	P_3	P_4
Education	2		✓	✓		
Household income per capita	3		✓			
Number of rooms per house-hold member	4			✓	✓	✓
Simultaneous Variables	P_i					
Malnutrition	1			✓	✓	
Diarrhea	2		✓			
Respiratory	3		✓			
Lagged Variables	P^a_{i-1}					
Low birth weight	1		✓			

Table 3–2. *(Continued)*

Infant Age Group Fatality Functions

Activity or Variable	Subscript Notation	Activities Involved	Malnutrition Only	Diarrhea Only	Respiratory Only	Inoculable Only	Malnutrition + Inoculable	Malnutrition + Diarrhea	Malnutrition + Respiratory	Other Combinations (2 + 3, 2 + 4, 3+ 1, 2 + 3 + 4)
Intervention Activities	I_i	X_i	f_1	f_2	f_3	f_4	f_5	f_6	f_7	f_8
Outpatient care	32	27		U_7	U_7	U_7	U_7	U_7	U_7	U_7
Inpatient care	33	28		U_7	U_7	U_7	U_7	U_7	U_7	U_7

Toddler Age Group Usage Functions

Activity or Variable	Subscript Notation	Activities Involved	Usage of Preventive Care	Usage of Curative Care
Intervention Activities	I_i	X_i	U_8	U_9
Promotora	1	1	✓	✓
Mass media	24	22	✓	✓
Well-baby clinic	34	29		✓
Socioeconomic Variables	S_i			
Household income	1		✓	✓
Education	2		✓	✓

Table 3–2. *(Continued)*

		Toddler Age Group Morbidity Functions				
Activity or Variable	*Subscript Notation*	*Activities Involved*	*Malnutrition*	*Diarrhea*	*Respiratory*	*Inoculable*
Intervention Variables	I_i	X_i	P_1	P_2	P_3	P_4
Promotora	1	1	✓			
Water: in home	20	18		✓		
public fountain	21	19		✓		
Sanitation: in house toilet	22	20		✓	✓	✓
latrines	23	21		✓	✓	✓
Immunization: DPT, polio, measles	27	23				U_6
Well-baby clinic	34	29	U_8	U_8	U_8	
Nutritional supp., child	35	30	U_8			
Socioeconomic Variables	S_i		P_1	P_2	P_3	P_4
Education	2		✓	✓		
Household income per household member	3		✓			
Number of rooms per household member	4			✓	✓	✓
Simultaneous Variables	P_i					
Malnutrition	1			✓	✓	✓
Diarrhea	2		✓			
Respiratory	3		✓			
Immunizable	4		✓		✓	
Lagged Variables	P_{i-1}					
Malnutrition	1		✓			

Table 3–2. *(Continued)*

			Toddler Age Group Fatality Functions							
Activity or Variable	*Subscript Notation*	*Activities Involved*	*Malnutrition Only*	*Diarrhea Only*	*Respiratory Only*	*Inoculable Only*	*Malnutrition + Inoculable*	*Malnutrition + Diarrhea*	*Malnutrition + Respiratory*	*Other Combinations (2 + 3, 2 + 4, 3+ 1, 2 + 3 + 4)*
Intervention Activities	I_i	X_i	f_1	f_2	f_3	f_4	f_5	f_6	f_7	f_8
Outpatient care	36	32		U_9	U_9	U_9	U_9	U_9	U_9	U_9
Inpatient care	37	31		U_9	U_9	U_9	U_9	U_9	U_9	U_9

Appendix 3A

A Note on the Specification of the Morbidity Functions

This appendix gives a derivation and algebraic interpretation of the functional form used for the morbidity equations. The explanation is given for the malnutrition equations and the specification of the other equations is asserted by analogy. The derivation is, by necessity, a simplification of a complex process and ignores certain features of the process to concentrate on the major aspects.

The specification proceeds by partitioning the total number of surviving children (N) into those who were malnourished in the previous period (N_m) and those who were well (N_w). Figure 3A–1 depicts this partitioning. The number who were well is partitioned into those who become malnourished in the present period (N_{wm}) and those who remain well (N_{ww}). The number who were malnourished is partitioned into those who remain malnourished (N_{mm}) because of a failure (attributed to physiological or noncontrol conditions) to adjust back to the norm and those who recover (N_{mw}) to standard weight (or would have recovered to standard weight if socioeconomic or intervention conditions would have permitted it). This latter number (N_{mw}) is further partitioned into the number of children who again become malnourished or who remain malnourished because of adverse control conditions and the number of previously malnourished children who recover and remain at standard weight (N_{mww}).

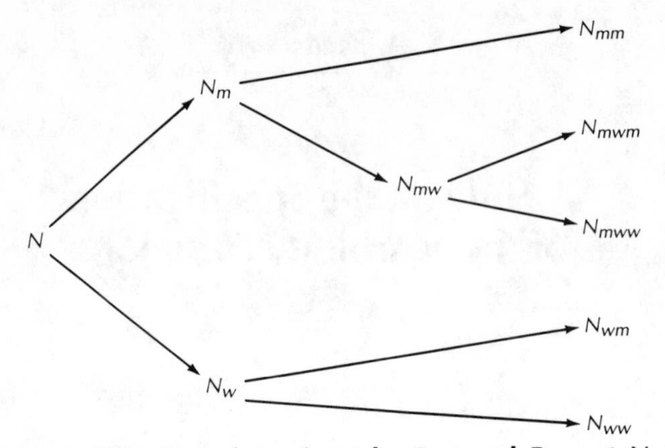

Figure 3A–1. Partitioning of Survivors by Past and Present Nutritional Status.

The key element in the partitioning is the conceptual distinction between children who were previously malnourished and could have recovered if socioeconomic and intervention (control) conditions had been favorable and previously malnourished children who remain malnourished because of adverse conditions and low levels of health interventions. The total (N'_{mm}) of these two categories of malnourished children is

$$N'_{mm} = N_{mm} + N_{mwm} \tag{3A–1}$$

and the number of malnourished children who fail to recover because of conditions beyond the control of the model is given by

$$N_{mm} = \gamma N_m \tag{3A–2}$$

where γ is the proportion of N_m who fail to recover because of an adverse health environment. In addition, presently malnourished children who were previously well are given by

$$N_{wm} = P^*_{1a} N_w \tag{3A–3}$$

where P^*_{1a} is the proportion of previously well children who become malnourished in the present (a) age group. Assuming this relationship is also approximately valid for N_{mwm} and N_{mw}, we write

$$N_{mwm} = P^*_{1a} N_{mw} \tag{3A–4}$$

Finally the number of previously malnourished children who could potentially recover in this age group is

$$N_{mw} = (1 - \gamma)N_m. \tag{3A–5}$$

Substituting (3A–2), (3A–3), and (3A–5) in (3A–1) and dividing the resulting equation by N_m gives an expression for the proportion of previously malnourished children surviving and malnourished in the present age group.

$$P'_{1a} = \gamma + P^*_{1a}(1 - \gamma) \quad \left(= \frac{N'_{mm}}{N_m}\right) \tag{3A–6}$$

The proportion of previously well children who become malnourished, P^*_{1a}, is a weighted average of the proportion caused by other diseases, P_j, and the proportion that is a logit function, $L_{1a}(I,S)$, of the level of interventions and socioeconomic variables. Let β_{ija} be the weight for the influence of the jth disease, then

$$P^*_{1a} = (1 - \sum_j \beta_{1ja}) \cdot L_{1a}(I,S) + \sum_j \beta_{1ja}P_{ja} \tag{3A–7}$$

The overall proportion of surviving children who are malnourished, P_{1a}, is a weighted average of P'_{1a} (equation 3A–6) and P^*_{1a} (equation 3A–7),

$$P_{1a} = \rho P'_{1a} + (1 - \rho)P^*_{1a}$$

where the weight, ρ, is the proportion of all survivors who were previously malnourished. Substituting from equations (3A–7) and (3A–6) yields,

$$P_{1a} = (1 - \gamma\rho) \cdot (1 - \sum_j \beta_{1ja}) \cdot L_{1a}(I,S) + (1 - \gamma\rho) \cdot \sum_j \beta_{1ja}P_{ja} + \gamma\rho \tag{3A–8}$$

In application, both γ and ρ are small enough fractions so that $\gamma\rho$ has a negligible influence on P_{1a} when multiplied by β_{1ja} *or* $L(I,S)$, which are also fractions. After (1) dropping $\gamma\rho$ from the first two terms; (2) adding the condition that the sum of the coefficients equal unity; and (3) substituting P_{1a-1}, the proportion of children malnourished in the previous age group (as an approximation of ρ), equation (3A–8) becomes the morbidity function used to model malnutrition in the last two age groups.

$$P_{1a} = a_{1a} \cdot L_{1a}(I,S) + \sum_j b_{1ja}P_{ja} + c_{1a}P_{1a-1} \tag{3A–9}$$

where $a_{1a} = (1 - \sum_j \beta_{1ja} - c_{1a})$, $b_{1ja} = \beta_{1ja}$, *and* $c_{1a} = \gamma$. With the omission of the lagged relationship equation (3A–8) becomes the morbidity function used for all other marginal morbidity rates,

$$P_{ia} = a_{ia} \cdot L_{ia}(I,S) + \sum_j b_{ija} P_{ja} \qquad \text{(3A–10)}$$

where $a_{ia} = 1 - \sum b_{ija}$.

Chapter 4

The Community and Baseline Data

INTRODUCTION

To allow an operâtional application of the morbidity-mortality model, baseline data describing a hypothetical community was assembled. By delimiting the population, initial disease prevalence, mortality rates, and the initial availability of health services, the baseline data sets the scale of the analysis and the potential improvement in the objective. A realistic setting is provided by choosing baseline values that are consistent with the health environment for a marginal low-income, urban area in Cali, Colombia.

The area described in the analysis approximates five barrios in Cali—Antonio Narino, El Diamente, Union de Vivenda Popular, Mariamos Ramos, and Republica de Israel. In 1968 the community was largely comprised of recent migrants. Only a negligible proportion of households had intradomiciliary water; a large proportion of households were located near open sewage. Much of the housing was temporary with dirt floors and roads were unpaved. Water was located at a significant distance from households or was vended periodically from trucks. Health institutions were poorly and sporadically used. Data gathered in 1973 indicate that 18 percent of the work force was unemployed or underemployed in marginal part-time occupations.[1]

Although the area selected is now the focus of attention for several experimental health programs, most notably the PRIMOPS project,[a] these programs were not in existence prior to 1970. The baseline morbidity and health activity data are intended to apply to the community as it was in the period from 1968 to 1970 and prior to the recent experimental health interventions. Because accurate data does not exist prior to 1970, the baseline morbidity data is derived from an extrapolation of preliminary data gathered between 1973 and 1976 as part of the PRIMOPS project and from analogies with similar populations in other studies. Ultimately baseline data deficiencies were severe enough that several rates had to be chosen arbitrarily and, for this reason, we emphasize that the community should be regarded as hypothetical and only an approximation of a low-income community in Cali, Colombia.

POPULATION AND SOCIOECONOMIC DATA

While the socioeconomic data are intended to apply to the community prior to 1970, the population data, which determine the scale of the resources needed, are estimates for 1976. The role of the socioeconomic variables in the morbidity and usage functions is as an index and the scale of the variables only serves to determine the scale of the coefficients. In contrast, the role of the population data is to determine the scale or absolute level of health activities needed to achieve a given percentage of coverage. For this reason, the population data are coordinated with the data of the enumeration of available resources. Baseline population and socioeconomic data are given in Table 4–1. The subscripts refer to the subscripts of the socioeconomic variables in the morbidity equations in the text and in the computer program in the appendix. Additional baseline population data are given in Table 6–15 in Chapter 6.

BASELINE MORBIDITY AND MORTALITY RATES

The baseline morbidity rates (see Table 4–2) are estimated from unpublished data and preliminary reports of the PRIMOPS project.[2] The rates are marginal morbidity rates, that is, they represent the proportion

[a] The PRIMOPS project (Programa de Investigacion en Modelos de Prestacion de Servicios de Salud) was established as a joint project of the Colombian ministry of health, the state of Valle, and the University of Valle. The objective of the project is to provide a set of coordinated health services for women of childbearing age and children. The services are similar to those being considered in this analysis. A more complete description of the program is given in César Corzantes, "Synthesis of 'Primops' Technical Background Material," and Jaime Rodrigues and Jesus Rico, *Componentes Evaluativos.*

Table 4–1. Baseline Population Data and Socioeconomic Data.

I. Population Data			*Source*
Total population		69,110	Marnane
Number of families		12,319	Marnane
Number of women 15–49		15,412	Marnane
Children 0–4 years of age		12,713	Marnane
0–1 years of age		2,903	Marnane
1–4 years of age		9,810	Marnane
Average family size		5.6	Marnane
II. Socioeconomic Data	S_i		
Average household income (US$)	1	580	Corzantes
Proportion of household heads with four or more years of education	2	.30	Estimate based on data from Corzantes
Income per household member (US$)	3	104	Corzantes, Marnane
Proportion of households with less than 2 people per room	4	.20	Estimate based on unpublished data
Proportion of women exposed to pregnancy[a] who are			
between ages 18 and 35	5	.60	Santemaria and Daza
at risk of a birth with less than 2-year interval	6	.55	Santemaria and Daza

Sources: Patrick Marnane, "Primops Background Information, Community Profile of the U.V.P. Area," PRIMOPS document (mimeograph, Tulane University, School of Public Health, August 1977). César Corzantes, "Synthesis of 'Primops' Technical Background Material, Report A: Summary of 'Primops' Program" (mimeograph, Tulane University, School of Public Health, February 17, 1975). Alfonso Santemaria and Luis Daza, *Investigacion de Riesgo Materno-Infantil*, PRIMOPS document, Bogota, Colombia, 1977.

[a] This is the proportion of women who are married and not using a contraceptive method. These data are corroborated by estimates of the birth histories of mothers given in Jaime Rodriguez and Jesus Rico, eds., *Componentes Evaluativos de la Atencion Primaria*, PRIMOPS document, Cali, Colombia, 1977.

of the population having the disease irrespective of whether or not another disease is present. An attempt has been made to use disease definitions that are consistent with the survey questions and model specification. Malnutrition refers to grades II and III according to the Gomez classification and Diarrhea refers to cases classified as acute or severe. The rates for immunizable diseases are estimated by implication from mortality rates for the Cali area and from the Puffer and Serrano study.[3] The rate for neonatal tetanus is arbitrary and is included only to provide a realistic assessment of the contribution of trained midwife and institutional deliveries in an urban setting.[4]

Upper and lower bounds for the morbidity rates were set after a search of the literature and were made with reference to studies in areas as diverse as India, Guatemala, Haiti, the United States, and Britain; but the

Table 4–2. Baseline Morbidity Rates Used in the Specification of the Morbidity Functions.

	Upper Bound	Lower Bound	Baseline Rate in Five Barrio Populations
I. Neonatal Age Group			
Low birth weight	.30	.02	.10
Infection	.40	.04	.15
Birth trauma	.10	.02	.04
Tetanus	.30	.00	.005
Mortality rate/birth			.045
II. Infant Age Group			
Malnutrition (grades II & III)	.30	.00	.10
Diarrhea (severe)	.30	.00	.17
Lower respiratory	.10	.00	.06
Immunizable diseases	.06	.00	.005
Mortality rate per child in age group			.00513
III. Early Childhood			
Malnutrition (grades II & III)	.30	.00	.15
Diarrhea (severe)	.30	.00	.11
Lower respiratory	.10	.00	.02
Immunizable diseases	.04	.00	.004
Mortality rate per child in age group			.00117

Note: All rates are per 28-day period.

selection, especially of the upper bound, is ultimately arbitrary. Sensitivity tests with the final model reveal that the results are not greatly affected by ±33-percent changes in the upper bound as long as the value chosen is consistent[b] with the algebraic specification.

The twenty-eight-day mortality rates are based on estimates arrived at by comparison with similar communities elsewhere. Some guidance was provided by the data published in Puffer and Serrano,[5] although for most of the communities covered by that study the data refer to a sample of larger metropolitan areas and the rates are much lower than would generally be expected for lower-income subsamples.[c] The baseline mortality rates in Table 4–2 can be expressed in more familiar terms; the neonatal mortality rate is 45 per 1000 births (40 per 1000 without tetanus), the 1–12 month rate is 57 per 1000 births, and the early childhood rate is 55 per 1000 children aged one to four. The infant mortality rate (0–12 months) is 96 per 1000 births. Table 4–3 gives a further breakdown of the twenty-eight-day

[b] See p. 110 in Chapter 5.

[c] The Recife and San Juan samples do appear to be more homogeneous and we have used these samples later in Chapter 7 to check the reasonableness of the distribution of mortality rates produced by the simulation model.

Table 4–3. Calculation of Unexplained Mortality Rates.

Age Group	*Proportion of Total Mortality Explained By Diseases in Model*[a]	*Mortality Rate per 28-Day Period*[b]	*Rate of Explained Mortality*	*Rate of Unexplained Mortality*
	(col. 2)	(col. 3)	(col. 4 = col. 2 × col. 3)	(ψ_a)
0–1	.83	.04000	.03320	.00680
1–12	.83	.00513	.00426	.00087
12–60	.80	.00117	.00094	.00023

[a] Based on data from Ruth Puffer and Carlos Serrano, eds., *Patterns of Mortality in Childhood*, Pan American Health Organization, Scientific Publication No. 262, Washington, D.C., 1973. A midpoint of the Cali, San Juan, and Recife samples was taken. Disease definitions were interpreted loosely to conform to the definitions used in the model. Tetanus is not included.

[b] Based on assumed mortality rates of 40/1000 births for neonatal mortality, 60/1000 infants for the 1–12 month period, and 55/1000 children one-to-four years of age for the early childhood period.

mortality rates into the mortality explained by the diseases in the model and an unexplained residual. In the simulation model, the unexplained residual, ψ_a, is added to the mortality explained by the morbidity and fatality equations in each age group to obtain the final mortality rate used to generate the number of survivors. The unexplained rates remain unaltered throughout the simulation and optimization experiments.

BASELINE INTERVENTION RATES

Baseline intervention rates are given in Table 4–4. The subscripts in the table refer to the subscripts in the equations in the text and in the computer program in the appendix. The data are approximate and are based on the recollection of researchers and administrators working in the study area. The division of prenatal services into early and late recipients is based on a subjective estimate. The indefinite nature of the baseline intervention rates is underlined by the fact that the interventions available in 1968–1970 were only approximations of the more formally designed programs being considered by the cost-effectiveness model. Besides providing a description of the initial health services environment, the rates are used in the morbidity functions to provide an algebraic reference point in the conversion of survey responses to coefficients. Generally, the higher the baseline intervention rate the lower will be the coefficient in the morbidity function. However, the rates are uniformly low and sensitivity tests confirmed that the relative importance of various coefficients

Table 4–4. Baseline Intervention Rates.

Intervention	Subscript	Baseline Rate	Intervention	Subscript	Baseline Rate
PROMOTER	1	.00	H2OWALK	21	.50
AWTXINF	2	.01	TOILET	22	.10
AFEDEFTX	3	.01	LATRINE	23	.50
AWTXANE	4	.00	MMEDIA	24	.00
PWTXINF 2	5	.09	1 OUTP	25	.15
PWNUTLBW 2	6	.00	1 INP	26	.05
PWTETIMM 2	7	.26	IMMDPTPM	27	.10
PWHCED 2	8	.09	2 WBC	28	.10
PWNUT 2	9	.00	2 NUTCH	29	.00
DELINLBW	10	.05	2 BFWSUP	30	.00
PWTXINF 1	11	.01	2 BFNOSUP	31	.30
PWNUTLBW 1	12	.00	2 OUTP	32	.18
PWTETIMM 1	13	.04	2 INP	33	.02
PWHCED 1	14	.01	3 WBC	34	.10
PWNUT 1	15	.00	3 NUTCH	35	.00
DELIN	16	.05	3 OUTP	36	.18
DELMW	17	.15	3 INP	37	.02
DEL & PROM	18	.00			
BF	19	.30			
H2OHOME	20	.10			

Note: This is an approximate decription of 1968 rates, expressed as a proportion of the population covered by the intervention.

has not been greatly distorted by possible misspecification of these rates.[d]

NOTES

1. A number of documents give more descriptive information than can be included here. See César Corzantes, "Synthesis of 'Primops' Technical Background Material, Report A: Summary of 'Primops' Program" (mimeograph, Tulane University, School of Public Health, February 17, 1975); Jaime Rodriguez and Jesus Rico, eds., *Componentes Evaluativos de la Atençiòn Primaria*, PRIMOPS document, Cali, Colombia, 1977; Alfonso Santemaria and Luis Daza, *Investigacion de Riesgo Materno-Infantil*, PRIMOPS document, Bogota, Colombia, 1977; Patrick Marnane, "Primops Background Information, Community Profile of the U.V.P. Area," PRIMOPS document (mimeograph, Tulane University, School of Public Health, August 1977).

[d] Note in equation 5A–9 of Appendix 5A that the baseline intervention rate is added to one in the denominator. When the baseline rate is a very small fraction, changes in the rate have little impact on the calculated coefficient.

2. The data were assembled by Gildardo Agudelo of the PRIMOPS project. Supplemental data can be found in Arnold Levine, "Final Analysis of Health Post Record System Survey," PRIMOPS document (mimeograph, Tulane University, School of Public Health, October 1975); Beatrice Selwyn, "Further Analysis of Health Posts Record System Survey," PRIMOPS document (mimeograph, Tulane University, School of Public Health, July 12, 1975); Department of National Planning, "Distribución de las Poblacion en Estados de Salud Segun Cuasa, Edad Y Sexo," Bogota, Colombia, November 15, 1974; and Rodriguea and Rico, *Componentes Evaluativos.*
3. Ruth Puffer and Carlos Serrano, eds., *Patterns of Mortality in Childhood,* Pan American Health Organization, Scientific Publication No. 262, Washington, D.C., 1973.
4. A strong case for the importance of neonatal tetanus in the absence of hygienic deliveries or maternal immunization is made by Warren L. Berggren and Gretchen M. Berggren, "Changing Incidence of Fatal Tetanus in the Newborn," *American Journal of Tropical Medicine and Hygiene* 20 (1971): 491–494; and G. B. Simmons, C. Smucker, B. D. Misra, and P. Majumdar, "Patterns and Causes of Infant Mortality in Rural Uttar Pradesh," *Journal of Tropical Pediatrics and Child Health* (October 1978): 207–216.
5. Puffer and Serrano, *Patterns of Mortality.*

Chapter 5

Specification of the Structural Parameters of the Child Mortality Model

INTRODUCTION

The model described in Chapter 4 is intended to involve the minimum number of relationships necessary for the specification of a quantitative planning model to be used for the evaluation of policy choices affecting child mortality. An effort was made to include only the most important disease relationships and the most feasible interventions from among the host of interrelationships and interventions that might be identified. The goal was to keep the model tractable while still being large enough to provide a practical illustration of the construction of a disease model for cost-effectiveness analysis. This effort notwithstanding, there is still a total of 221 parameters (coefficients) that need to be specified before the model can be applied. Potentially, the parameters could be specified statistically using data from field studies and clinical research. In fact, the parameters provide a catalogue of the separate problem areas that have been the focus of medical and health research on child mortality in developing regions over the last twenty to thirty years. However, in spite of the substantial body of operational and theoretical research on the treatment and prevention of childhood disease, the extant literature does not allow the complete specification of the quantitative relationships required by even the modest dimensions of the child mortality simulation model. The major problem with

Table 5–1. Number of Parameters to be Specified in the Structural Equations.

Equation Type	Age Group	Number of Parameters	
Usage	Neonatal	20	
	Infant	10	
	Toddler	10	
		Subtotal	40
Morbidity	Neonatal	52	
	Infant	29	
	Toddler	28	
		Subtotal	109
Fatality	Neonatal	24	
	Infant	24	
	Toddler	24	
		Subtotal	72
		Total	221

an objective specification of the model is that the results of existing studies are not always summarized in the required quantitative form and even when the research is sufficiently explicit from a quantitative standpoint, it is based on controlled experimental conditions or is derived from disparate economic, social, and physical environments that are not replicated in the area being analyzed in this study. Further, the cost of an objective study large enough to yield estimates of all the parameters in the model would have carried us beyond the scale of the present project both in time and money.

For these reasons, we decided to specify the parameters through the use of a set of survey questions designed for that purpose. An advantage of the survey procedure is that it allows the opinion of medical and health practitioners with considerable experience in the problems of delivering health services in less developed countries to be utilized in the specification of the model's parameters in the context of an actual environment in a specific location. Ultimately, survey results should be compared and supplemented, where possible, with the results from statistical analyses of usage, morbidity, and fatality data under various intervention conditions. An argument can be made, however, that given the tremendous statistical and conceptual problems that are faced in experimental research, a subjective specification derived from the opinions of people who have first-hand experience is a more applicable and accurate method for the specification of a practical optimization model at the present time.

It is apparent that the quality, rather than the number of survey participants is important for this study. Given the budget and time restriction, we decided to limit the survey to sixteen health professionals of outstanding reputations. Of this number, ten were from Colombia, the country in which the community being analyzed is located, and six were chosen internationally. Survey participants were selected from a number of different fields—maternal and perinatal health, nutrition, environmental sanitation, pediatrics, and epidemiology. The participants also differed from the point of view of institutional affiliation and experience and included medical doctors, public health specialists, and scientists engaged in the selection and administration of government or institutional health policies, the actual delivery of medical and health services, and research related to the estimation of health intervention effectiveness and interdisease relationships.

The survey consisted of four different sets of questions covering, respectively, usage, morbidity, fatality, and disease interactions. Respondents were asked questions appropriate to their experience and knowledge, with no respondent asked the total of all four sets of questions. Table 5–2 gives the number of respondents included in each category.

All participants were asked the morbidity questions. The disease interaction questions were asked primarily of institutional researchers who have been involved in studying the interaction between malnutrition and infection. The questions concerning fatality rates were asked of health professionals with clinical experience. Finally the survey questions with regard to usage were asked only of Colombian respondents. This is because the effects of alternative policies and socioeconomic variables on participation rates are apt to be determined by institutions, traditions, and customs that are particular to the study area. In contrast the other sets of questions involve relationships that have strong physiological bases that are likely to be independent of the area under analysis.

The survey was conducted in personal interviews each of which took approximately one day to complete.[a] A number of comments were received

[a] It is emphasized that participation does not imply any agreement with the results of this study. We are very grateful for the generous cooperation of: Alfredo Aguirre, PRIMOPS project (director), Cali; Edgar Cobo, Universidad del Valle; William Cutting, London School of Hygiene and Tropical Medicine; Luis Fajardo, Proyecto de Nutricion, Universidad del Valle; Jean-Pierre Habicht, Division of Nutritional Sciences, Cornell University; A. Herrera, Universidad del Valle; James Koopman, School of Public Health, University of Michigan; David Morley, Institute of Child Health, University of London; Alberto Pradilla, World Health Organization, New Delhi; Hernando Rey, Universidad del Valle; Jaime Rodriguez, PRIMOPS project (former director), Cali; Alfonso Santemaria, Antioquia University; F. M. Shattock, Liverpool School of Tropical Medicine and Hygiene; A. Tafur, Universidad del Valle; Ronald Wilson, DEIDS/Lampang Development Project, Thailand; and Joe D. Wray, Harvard School of Public Health.

Table 5–2. Number of Survey Participants by Category of Survey Frame.

	Survey Frame			
	Usage	Morbidity	Disease Interaction	Fatality
Colombian participants	8	10	3	6
Non-Colombian participants	–	6	3	2
	8	16	6	8

Note: The totals are not additive because some survey participants answered questions from more than one survey frame.

with regard to specific responses and in many cases the comments resulted in modifications to the final simulation model or in qualifications that we have attempted to incorporate in the interpretation of results. All participants recognized that a survey of opinion is only a stopgap procedure and must ultimately be replaced by objective scientific analysis. Participation took place in the spirit of professional inquiry and a search for a solution to the pressing problem of child mortality. It is to be noted that the results reported here do not necessarily represent the opinion of any participant individually.

All questions were answered under the assumption that the program or activity being considered has been operating for a long enough period to achieve a stable (or equilibrium) impact on the population in question. Also, each question assumes that all other programs and conditions are remaining unchanged except for the activity under consideration.

ESTIMATES OF THE IMPACT OF HEALTH INTERVENTIONS ON CHILD MORBIDITY

Response Format

In general, the morbidity questions were asked in the form of elasticities, that is, the questions were designed to give the percentage change in one variable (for instance, the rate of neonatal infections) in response to a percentage change in another (for instance, the percentage of children delivered in a health center). The primary advantage of an elasticity is that it can be estimated without knowledge of the units of measurement. A second advantage of the use of elasticities is that the estimates can be related to a variety of functional forms without requiring an additional survey. Appendix 5A gives the algebraic relationship between the survey responses and the morbidity functions used in the child mortality model.

Preliminary tests with the questionnaires showed that there is no one method of response that would be satisfactory for all participants or for all questions. For this reason a variety of procedures were devised, and the format of the response tables was designed accordingly, so that the question and response format with which each participant felt the most comfortable could be used. In order of desirability, from the point of view of specifying the model, the procedures were: (1) a subjective point estimate; (2) an 80 percent confidence range; and (3) a subjective response on a scale of one to ten. Fortunately, most respondents felt comfortable with the first two procedures, which yield answers that are more readily translated into impact coefficients than are the answers derived from the latter procedure. Explanations of the three procedures and the use of the response tables are provided here.

Point Estimate: Respondents were asked to give their subjective estimate of the percentage change in the morbidity rate among 100 new recipients of the intervention under consideration.

Range: Respondents were asked to give an interval for the percentage change in the morbidity rate among 100 new recipients that has, approximately, an 80 percent chance of containing the true percentage change.

Scale: Using a scale, respondents were asked to choose the number between one and ten that best conveys their opinion of the impact of the intervention on the reference population.

Confidence in Answers

The degree of confidence the respondent places in his answer was obtained for all morbidity responses. Confidence may fluctuate with variations in the fields of specialization of the participants and in the extent of contemporary knowledge about particular interventions and relationships. For instance, wide fluctuations in the confidence placed in the responses to a particular question might reflect a respondent panel made up of people who have extensively researched a given relationship as well as people who have little familiarity with the relationship. In contrast, a low degree of confidence among all responding to a given question might indicate that, with the present state of knowledge, little is known about the relationships needed to answer the question. Confidence is measured on a scale of zero to five as defined in Table 5–3.

Participants were forewarned that most of the questions require subjective estimates and in many cases the estimates may be no more than "educated" quesses. However, it was emphasized that even though hard

Table 5–3. Scale for Confidence in Accuracy of Answers.

0	Can't answer this question.
1	Not highly confident, but an educated guess is possible.
2	Somewhat confident. No hard data are available but clinical or field experience allows a guess.
3	Moderately confident. Although some controversy may exist, there is tentative support based on data and/or a consensus of practitioners with clinic or field experience would support this estimate.
4	Confident. Personal knowledge through extensive research or clinical and field experience leads to this estimate; controversy is minimal.
5	Highly confident. This estimate is the accepted professional opinion and can be considered incontrovertible at the present time.

data are lacking and controversy may exist, a response is important if it is based, intuitively or otherwise, on clinical, field, or research knowledge.

Summary of Morbidity Responses

The difficulty in making subjective estimates of the impact of health interventions is underscored by the substantial variability in the responses to the morbidity survey frame. Table 5–4 gives subjective estimates of the proportional reduction in morbidity rates, in specified reference populations, for the various interventions being considered by the child morbidity model. The values reported represent the averages of all responses obtained for a given intervention. The variability of the responses is illustrated by the large standard deviations that range from one-third to twice the value of the mean estimates. The speculative character of the responses is also indicated by the modest (although not low) level of the confidence in the responses; for most interventions the participants indicated that they were slightly to moderately confident in their responses and that the responses ranged from guesses based on field experience to conclusions derived from tentative data. It is clear from the variability in the responses and from the modest level of confidence given that the impact estimates should be applied circumspectly.

The average responses do, however, exhibit a qualitative consistency with the literature in those cases where tentative objective data are available, and a comparison of responses to alternative interventions reveals that they retain an internal consistency as well. For example, the largest impacts on infant diarrhea and neonatal infection are predicted to be made by breast feeding. This correlates well with a number of studies that indicate the dramatic effect of breast feeding in reducing infant diarrhea.[1] Similarly, estimates of the importance of age and birth interval for birth weight indicate that the subjective estimates are within an acceptable range of reported results.

An examination of Table 5–4 reveals patterns of responses for various categories of interventions. The direct, educational impact of the promotora intervention is seen as moderate but significant (approximately 0.17–0.20) for low birth weight, neonatal infection, and diarrhea in both infants and early childhood and somewhat higher for malnutrition (approximately 0.25–0.30). Since the promotora program is expected to affect the morbidity rate for a number of different diseases and age groups, the aggregate effect on mortality is potentially substantial. Other educational programs are consistently predicted to have substantially smaller impacts (0.10–0.12) on all diseases considered.

Prenatal care programs are predicted to have an impact on low birth weight that ranges from a low of 0.12 for iron fortification to 0.28 for a nutritional program for pregnant women. The impact of prenatal exams on infection is modest (0.13–0.16) and for most of the prenatal programs the high variability of the responses and of the confidence level indicated that, although the programs are potentially valuable, there is insufficient information to make a clear judgement of the impacts.

Nutritional programs were clearly assessed as having important impacts on low birth weight (0.23) and malnutrition (0.38 for a nutritional program covering 1–12 month old children and 0.39 for a program covering early childhood). Moreover, the estimates for the nutritional programs were given with a notably higher level of confidence. Taken together, nutritional programs and breast feeding would be expected to reduce a substantial proportion of malnutrition in infants. Respondents placed considerable confidence in this expectation, with the average response indicating that tentative data would support this conclusion.

Sizable impacts were also assigned to the effect of water and sanitary programs on diarrhea. The effects of water availability were seen as more important than sanitation with the effect of in-house piped water being considerably greater and assessed with more confidence than the effect of public fountains. The impact of extending water and sanitation coverage on those already having the interventions was seen as substantially less than the direct effects of the interventions. Nevertheless, the external effects of the water and sanitation interventions are not negligible and are generally at least 25 percent of the direct effects.

In contrast to the high level of confidence placed in the assessment of the impacts of water and sanitation on diarrhea, the estimates of the impacts of all of the interventions considered for respiratory diseases were made with relatively low levels of confidence. The interventions considered were also seen to have smaller discernible effects on respiratory diseases. Sanitary interventions are estimated to reduce the morbidity rate for lower respiratory diseases directly by only 0.01 to 0.02 in 12–60 month old children and by only 0.04 to 0.07 in 1–12 month old children. The indirect effects are

Table 5–4. Subjective Estimates of the Impact of Health Interventions on Child Morbidity (average responses).

Age Group (Months)	Disease	Intervention Description	I_i	Reference Population
0–1	Low birth weight	promotora—hygiene and nutritional ed.	1	presently without intervention
		health center—hyg. and nut. ed., 1st trimester	14	presently without intervention
		health center—hyg. and nut. ed., 2nd trimester	8	presently without intervention
		educ. attainment of mother, at least 4 years	S_2	presently without intervention
		exam and tx for infection, etc., all women	2	presently without intervention
		prenatal exam and tx for infection, etc. in 1st trimester	11	presently without intervention
		prenatal exam and tx for infection, etc. in 2nd trimester	5	presently without intervention
		anemia tx for anemic women only	3	presently without intervention
		iron fortification for all women	4	presently without intervention
		nutritional program (prot., cal., iron) preg. women, 1st trimester	15	presently without intervention
		nutritional (prot., cal., iron), l.b.w. risk preg. women, 1st trimester	12	presently without intervention
		nutritional program (prot., cal., iron) preg. women, 2nd or 3rd trimester	9	presently without intervention
		nutritional (prot., cal., iron), l.b.w. risk preg nancies, 2nd or 3rd trimester	6	presently without intervention
		in-home pipe water	20	without intervention
			20*X*	already have intervention
		public fountain <100M	21	without intervention
			21*X*	already have intervention
		in-house toilet	22	without intervention
			22*X*	already have intervention

Intervention Coverage	Number of Responses	Proportional Change in Morbidity Rate		Confidence[a]	
		Mean Response	Standard Deviation	Mean	Standard Deviation
100 additional women	16	−.172	.156	2.4	1.0
100 additional women	16	−.130	.135	2.5	1.1
100 additional women	16	−.110	.086	2.8	1.1
100 additional women	14	−.117	.100	2.4	1.1
100 additional women	16	−.117	.115	2.9	1.3
100 additional women	16	−.225	.218	3.0	1.4
100 additional women	16	−.193	.176	3.0	1.4
100 additional women	15	−.118	.101	2.8	1.1
100 additional women	13	−.122	.111	2.5	1.2
100 additional women	16	−.278	.252	2.8	1.1
100 additional women	16	−.256	.225	2.7	1.0
100 additional women	16	−.231	.219	3.2	1.1
100 additional women	16	−.233	.193	3.1	1.0
increase from 50% to 100% of HH	15	−.058	.064	2.2	1.1
	13	−.009	.018	2.2	1.3
increase from 50% to 100% of HH	15	−.037	.048	2.2	1.1
	13	−.005	.014	2.3	1.2
increase from 50% to 100% of HH	14	−.057	.055	2.2	1.1
	12	−.028	.049	2.4	1.3

[a] See Table 5–3 for an explanation of the scale for confidence.

Table 5–4. *(Continued)*

Age Group (Months)	Disease	Intervention: Description	Intervention: I_i	Reference Population
		latrine	23	without intervention
			23X	already have intervention
		a doubling of household income per person	S_3	
		no mother of age <18 or >35 years	S_5	mothers <18 & >35 years
		no mother with <2 yrs. birth interval	S_6	mother <2 yrs. birth int.
0–1	Infection	promotora—hygienic and nutritional ed.	1	presently without intervention
		health center—hyg. and nut. ed., 2nd trimester	14	presently without intervention
		health center—hyg. and. nut. ed., 2nd trimester	8	presently without intervention
		exam and tx for infection, etc., all women	2	presently without intervention
		prenatal exam and tx for infection etc., in 1st trimester	11	presently without intervention
		prenatal exam and tx for infection, etc. in 2nd trimester	5	presently without intervention
		breast feeding	19	doesn't breast feed
		delivery in health center	16	unattended home del., no profilaxis, no tet. imm.
		delivery at home by midwife	17	unattended home del., no profilaxis, no tet. imm.
		unattended delivery at home, eye and cord later by promotora	18	unattended home del., no profilaxis, no tet. imm.
		in-home piped water	20	without intervention
			20X	already have intervention
		public fountain <100M	21	without intervention
			21X	already have intervention
		in-house toilet	22	without intervention
			22X	already have intervention

Intervention Coverage	Number of Responses	Proportional Change in Morbidity Rate: Mean Response	Proportional Change in Morbidity Rate: Standard Deviation	Confidence[a]: Mean	Confidence[a]: Standard Deviation
increase from 50% to 100% of HH	14	−.044	.052	2.2	1.1
	12	−.010	.017	2.4	1.4
100 additional women	15	−.147	.133	2.3	.9
100 additional women	14	−.163	.094	3.1	1.3
100 additional women	14	−.181	.133	3.5	.9
100 additional women	16	−.164	.131	2.7	1.0
100 additional women	16	−.108	.075	2.4	1.0
100 additional women	16	−.128	.084	2.6	1.1
100 additional women	16	−.128	.090	2.7	1.2
100 additional women	16	−.158	.144	2.8	1.1
100 additional women	16	−.144	.132	2.7	1.0
100 additional women	16	−.298	.176	3.3	1.0
100 additional women	16	−.240	.165	3.1	1.0
100 additional women	16	−.183	.121	2.9	1.0
100 additional women	16	−.091	−.095	2.7	1.1
increase from 50% to 100% of HH	16	−.207	.197	2.8	1.3
	12	−.040	.052	2.6	1.4
increase from 50% to 100% of HH	15	−.101	.127	2.6	1.0
	11	−.009	.016	2.7	1.3
	15	−.167	.128	2.8	1.0
	12	−.097	.169	2.5	1.1

[a] See Table 5–3 for an explanation of the scale for confidence.

Table 5–4. *(Continued)*

Age Group (Months)	*Disease*	*Intervention Description*	I_i	*Reference Population*
		latrine	23	without intervention
			23X	already have intervention
		doubling of household income per person	S_3	
		mothers education ≥ 4 years	S_2	ed. of mother ≤2 years
		≤2 people per room	S_4	presently ≥3 people per room
	Birth trauma	exam and treatment for preg. women, 1st trimester	11	presently without intervention
		delivery in health center	16	unattended home del. no profilaxis., no tet. imm.
		delivery at home by midwife	17	unattended home del., no profilaxis, no tet. imm.
		delivery of l.b.w. and b.t. risk mother in h.c.	10	unattended home del., no profilaxes, no tet. imm.
		no mother <18 or >35	54	mothers <18 & >35 years
		no mother with <2 birth interval	55	mother <2 yrs. birth int.
		exam and treatment in 2nd or 3rd trimester	5	presently without intervention
	Tetanus	delivery in health center	16	unattended home del., no profilaxis, no tet. imm.
		delivery at home by midwife	17	unattended home del., no profilaxis, no tet. imm.
		delivery unattended, a promotora visit later	18	unattended home del., no profilaxis, no tet. imm.
		prenatal hygienic education by promotora	1	presently without intervention
		prenatal hygienic education by health center	8 & 14	presently without intervention
1–12	Malnutrition	nutritional advice, promotora	1	presently without intervention
		nutritional advice, well-baby clinic	28	presently without intervention

Intervention Coverage	Number of Responses	Proportional Change in Morbidity Rate		Confidence[a]	
		Mean Response	Standard Deviation	Mean	Standard Deviation
increase from 50% to 100% of HH	15	−.116	.096	2.3	.8
	12	−.078	.138	2.1	.9
100 additional women	16	−.130	.120	2.4	1.2
100 additional women	16	−.096	.077	2.4	1.2
100 additional women	16	−.105	.102	2.5	1.2
100 additional women	16	−.172	.191	2.7	1.2
100 additional women	16	−.385	.228	3.0	1.2
100 additional women	16	−.187	.140	2.7	1.1
100 additional women	16	−.361	.225	2.9	1.3
100 additional women	15	−.210	.106	3.1	1.0
100 additional women	16	−.113	.133	2.8	1.5
100 additional women	16	−.209	.198	2.8	1.4
100 additional women	15	−.721	.269	4.1	.6
100 additional women	15	−.603	.283	3.8	.7
100 additional women	15	−.184	.257	3.1	1.0
100 additional women	15	−.241	.204	3.0	1.2
100 additional women	15	−.280	.272	3.0	1.2
100 additional children	14	−.240	.219	2.7	1.0
100 additional children	14	−.170	.159	2.7	.9

[a] See Table 5–3 for an explanation of the scale for confidence.

Table 5–4. *(Continued)*

Age Group (Months)	Disease	Intervention: Description	Intervention: I_i	Reference Population
		nutritional supplement, all children	29	presently without intervention
		breast feeding, no supplement	31	presently not breast feeding
		breast feeding with nutritional supplement for mother	30	breast feeding without supplement
		mothers education ≥4 years	S_2	ed. of mother ≤2 years
		doubling of household income per person	S_3	
	Diarrhea	in-home piped water	20	without intervention
			20X	already have intervention
		public fountain <100M	21	without intervention
			21X	already have intervention
		in-home excreta disposal	22	without intervention
			22X	already have intervention
		latrine	23	without intervention
			23X	already have intervention
		hygienic counsel, promotora	1	presently without intervention
		hygienic counsel, health clinic	28	presently without intervention
		ed. ≥4 years.	S_2	ed. of mother ≤2 years
		<2 people per room	S_4	presently 3 people per room
		breast feeding	31	doesn't breast feed
	Respiratory	in-house toilet	22	without intervention
			22X	already have intervention
		latrines	23	without intervention
			23X	already have intervention
		hygienic education, health center	28	presently without intervention
		breast feeding	31	doesn't breast feed
		≤2 people per room	S_4	presently 3 people per room
	Immunizable	breast feeding	31	presently not breast feeding
		≤2 people per room	S_4	presently 3 people per room

Intervention Coverage	Number of Responses	Proportional Change in Morbidity Rate: Mean Response	Proportional Change in Morbidity Rate: Standard Deviation	Confidence[a]: Mean	Confidence[a]: Standard Deviation
100 additional children	14	−.376	.246	3.1	.9
100 additional children	14	−.338	.210	3.3	1.0
100 additional children	14	−.329	.263	3.0	1.1
100 additional children	14	−.127	.101	2.6	1.0
100 additional children	14	−.239	.173	2.6	1.0
from present 50% to 100% of pop.	13	−.325	.262	3.5	1.2
	12	−.087	.096	3.0	1.1
from present 50% to 100% of pop.	13	−.156	.168	3.0	.8
	11	−.033	.051	2.6	1.1
from present 50% to 100% of pop.	14	−.220	.190	3.3	1.1
	12	−.113	.110	2.9	1.1
from present 50% to 100% of pop.	14	−.138	.146	2.8	.6
	13	−.068	.081	2.1	.7
100 additional children	14	−.195	.139	2.8	1.2
100 additional children	14	−.128	.075	2.6	1.1
100 additional children	14	−.114	.092	2.5	1.0
100 additional children	14	−.070	.081	2.3	1.2
100 additional children	14	−.362	.184	3.2	.9
from present 50% to 100% of pop.	14	−.073	.112	2.5	1.1
	10	−.002	.003	2.6	1.1
from present 50% to 100% of pop.	13	−.036	.065	2.5	1.1
	10	−.003	.003	2.5	1.1
100 additional children	13	−.122	.118	2.5	1.1
100 additional children	13	−.209	.161	3.0	1.0
100 additional children	14	−.199	.189	2.8	1.0
100 additional women	13	−.129	.155	2.7	1.0
100 additional women	14	−.188	.183	2.9	1.1

[a] See Table 5–3 for an explanation of the scale for confidence.

Table 5–4. *(Continued)*

Age Group (Months)	Disease	Intervention Description	I_i	Reference Population
12–60	Malnutrition	nutritional advice, promotora	1	presently without intervention
		nutritional advice, well-baby clinic	34	presently without intervention
		nutritional supplement, all children	35	presently without intervention
		mothers education ≥4 years	102	ed. of mother ≤2 years
		doubling of household income	103	
	Diarrhea	in-home piped water	20	without intervention
			20*X*	already have intervention
		public fountain <100M	21	without intervention
			21*X*	already have intervention
		in-house excreta disposal	22	without intervention
			22*X*	already have intervention
		latrine	23	without intervention
			23*X*	already have intervention
		hygienic counsel, promotora	1	presently without intervention
		hygienic counsel, health center	34	presently without intervention
		mother education ≥4 years	S_2	ed. of mother ≤of 2 years
		≤2 people per room	S_4	presently 3 people per room
	Respiratory	in-house toilet	22	without intervention
			22*X*	already have intervention
		latrines	23	without intervention
			23*X*	already have intervention
		hygienic education, health center	34	presently without intervention
		≤2 people per room	S_4	presently 3 people per room
	Immunizable	in-house toilet	22	without intervention
			22*X*	already have intervention
		latrine	23	without intervention
			23*X*	already have intervention
		≤2 people per room	S_4	presently 3 people per room

Intervention Coverage	Number of Responses	Proportional Change in Morbidity Rate		Confidence[a]	
		Mean Response	Standard Deviation	Mean	Standard Deviation
100 additional children	14	−.291	.189	2.7	.9
100 additional children	14	−.175	.207	2.7	.9
100 additional children	14	−.394	.281	3.1	.8
100 additional children	14	−.156	.139	2.8	.8
100 additional children	14	−.294	.169	2.8	.8
from present 50% to 100% of pop.	14	−.309	.269	3.3	.9
	11	−.077	.101	2.8	.9
from present 50% to 100% of pop.	14	−.161	.162	2.7	.9
	11	−.051	.094	2.3	1.0
from present 50% to 100% of pop.	14	−.278	.225	3.2	1.0
	11	−.074	.084	2.8	.9
from present 50% to 100% of pop.	14	−.198	.168	2.9	.8
	11	−.039	.064	2.8	1.0
100 additional children	12	−.198	.150	2.6	.8
100 additional children	13	−.133	.093	2.5	.7
100 additional children	13	−.142	.131	2.3	.5
100 additional children	14	−.101	.114	2.5	.8
from present 50% to 100% of pop.	6	−.018	.025	1.8	.8
	6	−.003	.003	2.0	.8
from present 50% to 100% of pop.	6	−.010	.020	1.8	.8
	6	−.003	.003	2.0	.8
100 additional children	6	−.085	.102	1.8	.8
100 additional children	5	−.270	.144	2.5	.6
from present 50% to 100% of pop.	12	−.092	.104	2.5	.9
	10	−.024	.047	2.0	1.2
from present 50% to 100% of pop.	12	−.056	.085	2.4	1.4
	10	.047	.015	2.8	1.5
100 additional children	13	.085	.112	2.6	.9

[a] See Table 5–3 for an explanation of the scale for confidence.

negligible. Given the low level of confidence in the estimates and the extremely small impacts, the responses indicate that respiratory diseases are not highly amenable to control and their consideration is not apt to be a decisive factor in determining the composition of programs to reduce child mortality. This accords well with actual practice where it is found that diarrhea, malnutrition, and immunizable diseases are the targets of most ongoing programs.

ESTIMATES OF THE IMPACT OF HEALTH INTERVENTIONS ON FATALITY

Estimates of case fatality rates for the joint disease categories considered by the model were obtained and included the fatality rate in the absence of formal care as well as the rates for outpatient or inpatient care. The actual responses were not used directly but were reformulated as relative fatality rates for the alternative disease states and types of care. The reason for this is that actual fatality rates vary greatly depending on the definition of morbidity, the degree of severity of the disease, the timing of the care, and the specific nature of the services provided. Because of the unknown variables involved, the absolute levels of the fatality rates obtained from the survey responses are difficult to interpret and there is no reason to expect that they will produce a level of mortality that will agree with the baseline data. Depending on the respondents' conceptions of these variables, the responses could, and did, vary greatly. In spite of the variation in the absolute level of responses, the relative magnitudes for the fatality rates across the disease states were fairly constant.

The relative magnitudes of the fatality rates were preserved[b] but the absolute levels were adjusted by rescaling the survey responses. This was done first by computing tentative baseline rates from a weighted average of the survey responses where the weights represented the baseline proportions of the population receiving each type of care. The tentative fatality rates were then used in conjunction with the baseline mortality and marginal morbidity rates given in Chapter 4, the estimates of the extent of disease interrelationships given in a subsequent section of this chapter, and the simulation model discussed in Chapter 3, to scale the absolute fatality rates. The procedure was to use the estimates of the marginal morbidity rates and interdisease relationships to produce a set of baseline joint disease rates. The tentative fatality rates (with the exception of tetanus for which the mean response was not altered) were then multiplied by a scaling factor chosen so that the resulting baseline fatality rates

[b] With the exception of the rates for the malnutrition and immunizable disease combination, which were adjusted upward by 0.25, and the neonatal rate for infection only, which was lowered by 0.5.

multiplied by the respective joint disease rate yielded the baseline mortality rate. Finally, the scaling factor was used to calculate rescaled no-care, outpatient, and inpatient rates.

An advantage of the procedure outlined above is that it preserves the opinions of the respondents with regard to the relative effectiveness of the different types of care in each of the disease states, and it produces mortality rates that are consistent with the baseline data. The distribution of mortality and the degree of accordance of the results of the procedure with the patterns of mortality noted in the PAHO study by Puffer and Serrano[2] are discussed in Chapter 7. Table 5–5 presents the resulting fatality rates. These rates differ from the actual mean responses by factors of 0.6, 0.6, and 0.2 for the neonatal, infant, and early childhood age groups. These factors represent the extent to which the unscaled responses overestimate the baseline mortality rates.

USAGE RESPONSE TO CHANGES IN SOCIOECONOMIC VARIABLES AND PROMOTIONAL INTERVENTIONS

The questions relating to program demand asked respondents to give estimates of the percentage of the relevant, eligible populations who would use specific categories of services before and after changes in related variables. The questions were asked alternatively under the assumption of present prices and the assumption that the services would be provided free of charge. At the present time, the charge for most of the services considered in the model is minimal and there was very little difference between the two sets of answers. These estimates were asked of participants who have been involved in various capacities in the delivery of health services in Cali in areas presently covered by promotional programs both before and after the programs were initiated. Appendix 5B gives the relationship between the survey responses and the coefficients in the usage functions.

Table 5–6 presents the mean responses for user demand at present prices; this is the data used in the simulations. The first column represents an estimate of the extent of the use of health services during the baseline period, 1968–1970. This estimate was made with reference to baseline data and does not come from survey responses. Similarly, the fourth row, which gives estimates of the proportion of women receiving prenatal care who receive care starting in the first trimester, is based on estimates of program administrators and not on the survey. The next five columns give the mean survey responses and indicate that in all usage categories the respondents consider the promotora program an extremely important means of increasing the use of health services, while the mass media programs, although effective, have a markedly smaller input on usage than does the

Table 5–5. Subjective Estimates of Fatality Rates for Joint Disease Categories (based on rescaled average responses).

I. 0–1 Month Age Group

	Tetanus (all states)	*Low Birth Weight Only*	*Birth Trauma Only*	*Infections Only*	*L.B.W. & B.T.*	*L.B.W. & inf.*	*B.T. & inf.*	*L.B.W. & B.T. & inf.*
No care	.910	.178	.230	.031	.350	.293	.293	.408
Outpatient	.874	.129	.202	.018	.292	.222	.235	.334
Inpatient	.448	.080	.124	.010	.185	.133	.142	.236

II. 1–12 Month Age Group

	Malnutrition Only	*Diarrhea Only*	*Respiratory Only*	*Immunizable Only*	*Maln. & Immun.*	*Maln. & Diarrhea*	*Maln. & Respiratory*	*Other Comb.*
No care	.006	.007	.014	.079	.154	.021	.026	.050
Outpatient	.004	.002	.006	.058	.111	.011	.015	.034
Inpatient	.002	.001	.003	.030	.060	.008	.010	.018

III. 12–60 Month Age Group

	Malnutrition Only	*Diarrhea Only*	*Respiratory Only*	*Immunizable Only*	*Maln. & Immun.*	*Maln. & Diarrhea*	*Maln. & Respiratory*	*Other Comb.*
No care	.0030	.0020	.0030	.0290	.0530	.0070	.0060	.0240
Outpatient	.0013	.0007	.0012	.0182	.0329	.0036	.0035	.0132
Inpatient	.0008	.0003	.0005	.0107	.0197	.0022	.0021	.0065

Table 5–6. Usage Response under Various Situations When Services Are Provided at the Present Nominal Prices (average of all respondents).

Usage Category	*Subscript Notation (U)*	*1968–1970 Baseline[a] Situation*	*Present (approx. in 1976)*	*A Doubling of Present Income*	*Increase in Average Educational Level of Mother to 4 Years*	*100% Coverage by Mass Media Program*	*100% Coverage by Health Promoter Program*
1. Prenatal care, all women	U_{11}	.10	.22	.32	.32	.49	.66
2. Prenatal care, pregnant women	U_{21}	.12	.24	.33	.43	.49	.75
3. Curative care, neonatal	U_{31}	.20	.20	.33	.30	.39	.63
4. Breast feeding	U_{41}	.30	.30	.30	.39	.47	.67
5. Prop. prenatal care in 1st trimester	U_{51}	.12	.12	.33	.40	.50	.75
6. Preventive care, infant	U_{12}	.10	.17	.26	.28	.37	.73
7. Curative care, infant	U_{22}	.20	.42	.45	.44	.54	.75
8. Preventive care, toddlers	U_{13}	.10	.17	.25	.31	.46	.76
9. Curative care, toddlers	U_{23}	.20	.43	.43	.46	.57	.69

[a] Estimates not based on survey responses.

promotora program. A significant aspect of the promotional programs is that they increase the use of preventive care relative to the use of curative care, especially in the infant and early childhood age groups. Initially, the proportion of the eligible participants using preventive services is less than half the proportion for curative care, but after 100 percent coverage by a promoter program, the participation rates are in approximate parity. While we must wait for the simulations to fully evaluate the impact of this fact, it is obvious that it at least raises the possibility that, by shifting demand to relatively less expensive preventive services, the level of morbidity will be sufficiently reduced that the pressure on curative care facilities will not be greatly increased even though the participation rate (for those needing the service) for curative care is also increased by the promotional programs.

THE EXTENT OF INTERDISEASE CAUSAL RELATIONSHIPS

This survey frame provided for a scale, a range, or a best estimate to be used as a response. The questions were intended to reveal the extent to which the presence of one disease is caused by another. The questions do not ask the extent to which disease X can be found in association with Y but, instead ask the extent to which having Y is attributable to having X. This allows the responses to be interpreted directly as the coefficients, b_{ija}, representing interdisease causal relationships in the morbidity equations (see Chapter 3). Given the linear form of the morbidity functions, the value of b_{ij} represents the proportion of the incidence of disease i that is explained by disease j, and one minus the sum of the b_{ij} for a given equation represents the proportion of disease i that can be influenced or eliminated through changes in interventions and socioeconomic conditions without a concommittant change in linked diseases. This arbitrary apportionment of the observed disease rate between the two sources of causes—other diseases and control conditions—is dependent on the linear form of the function and the omission of joint causal effects and interactive terms. Ultimately the extent of causal relationships should be examined statistically through the estimation of simultaneous functional forms.

Table 5–7 gives the mean value of the estimates of the proportion of disease A that will lead to disease B. The extent of variation across respondents is also indicated. The most important interdisease relationships noted are those between malnutrition and diarrhea. With a high degree of uniformity, respondents stated that severe diarrhea in infants was a highly important cause of malnutrition. The converse relationship, that of malnutrition leading to diarrhea, was also noted to be moderate to high but there was much less uniformity of opinion with regard to the relationship in the early childhood age group. Similarly there was variation

Table 5–7. Subjective Estimates of Interdisease Causal Relationships.

Age Group (Months)	*Disease*			*Coefficient Notation*[a]	*Estimated Coefficient*[b]	*Variation Among Respondents*
	A	*affects*	*B*			
0–1	low birth weight		infection	b_{121}	.21	high
1–12	diarrhea		malnutrition	b_{212}	.36	low[c]
1–12	respiratory		malnutrition	b_{312}	.07	low
1–12	malnutrition		diarrhea	b_{122}	.23	moderate
1–12	malnutrition		respiratory	b_{132}	.10	low
12–60	diarrhea		malnutrition	b_{213}	.38	low[c]
12–60	respiratory		malnutrition	b_{313}	.08	low
12–60	immunizable		malnutrition	b_{413}	.20[d]	high
12–60	malnutrition		diarrhea	b_{123}	.25	high
12–60	malnutrition		respiratory	b_{133}	.07	moderate
12–60	immunizable		respiratory	b_{433}	.23	high
12–60	malnutrition		immunizable	b_{143}	.01[d]	low

[a] The first subscript denotes disease *A*, the second disease *B*, and the third the age group.

[b] In the first one, for example, the coefficient can be read as 21 percent of l.b.w. cases result in infections.

[c] One respondent felt strongly that this relationship is negligible. The remaining participants consistently estimated the relationship to be important.

[d] Coefficient b_{413} was arbitrarily reduced from 0.33 to 0.20 and coefficient b_{413} was reduced from 0.04 to 0.01 to meet the algebraic consistency requirements for the equations. See Appendix 5A for a discussion of the consistency requirements.

in the opinion of the extent of the causal relationship between low birth weight and neonatal infection.

Another moderately high causal relationship, also with a high degree of variation among the respondents, was that leading from immunizable diseases to malnutrition. However, because the baseline attack rate for immunizable diseases is low while the rate of malnutrition is high, the causal relationship flowing from immunizable diseases to malnutrition is not an important component in explaining the rate of malnutrition. On the other hand, although the degree of causal relationship flowing from malnutrition to immunizable diseases is low, the disparity in the attack rates implies that a high rate of malnutrition can be a significant factor in determining the rate of immunizable diseases.

NOTES

1. See, for example, Joe D. Wray, "Maternal Nutrition, Breast-Feeding and Infant Survival," in *Nutrition and Human Reproduction*, ed., W. Henry Mosley (New York: Plenum Press, 1978).
2. Ruth Puffer and Carlos Serrano, eds., *Patterns of Mortality in Childhood*, Pan American Health Organization, Scientific Publication No. 262, Washington, D.C., 1973.

Appendix 5A

Specification of the Coefficients in the Morbidity Functions

Referring to equation (3A–9) in Appendix 3A, the equation of a morbidity function for age group (a) can be written

$$P_{ia} = a_{ia} \cdot L_{ia}(I, S) + \sum b_{ija} P_{ja} + c_{ia} P_{ia-1} \qquad (5A\text{–}1)$$

where
$$L_{ia}(I, S) = \frac{\alpha_{iaU}}{1 + e^{-Z_{ia}}} + \alpha_{iaL}$$

and
$$Z_{ia} = \alpha_{oia} + \sum_k \alpha_{kia} I_k + \sum_l \alpha_{lia} S_l$$

COEFFICIENTS a, b, c

Given an estimate of the adjustment coefficient, (c_{ia}) and estimates of the interaction coefficients (b_{ija}) based on the survey responses, the weight (a_{ia}) on the intervention term can be calculated from the restriction that the sum of the linear weighting coefficients equals one, that is, $a_{ia} = 1 - \sum_j b_{ija} - c_{ia}$.

It will be recalled from Appendix 3A that $c_{ia} = \gamma$, which can be interpreted as the proportion of low-birth-weight or malnourished children who fail to recover to a weight of grade I or above even under optimum conditions. An algebraic expression for c_{ia}, in terms of parameters that are potentially observable, can be obtained by solving equation 3A–6 (in appendix to Chapter 3) for γ,

$$c_{ia} = \gamma_{ia} = \frac{P'_{ia} - P^*_{ia}}{1 - P^*_{ia}}$$

where P'_{ia} is the proportion of children malnourished (or low birth weight) in the previous period who remain malnourished in the present period and P^*_{ia} is the proportion of well children in the previous period who become malnourished in the present period. Baseline data were insufficient to allow a direct estimate of c_{ia}; as an alternative the coefficient was set arbitrarily and the model was examined for its sensitivity to the value of this coefficient after obtaining some idea of its magnitude by referring to data from other sources.

Using data giving the growth histories of a sample of children in the United States[a] to provide estimates of P'_{ia} and P^*_{ia}, the adjustment coefficient between low birth weight and malnourishment by the end of the first year (c_{12}) was approximately 0.1 while the coefficient relating malnourishment in the infant and early childhood age groups was 0.3. These estimates, especially the latter value of 0.3, are apt to be high, because a higher proportion of low-for-date weights in the United States are likely to be attributable to nonenvironmental physiological causes than in Colombia, but they do give an indication of the rate of adjustment under favorable conditions. Some indication that the latter coefficient is roughly of the correct magnitude was provided by a consideration of a small sample for Candelaria, Colombia,[1] which showed that after twelve months of participation in a nutritional program only 20 percent of children who were originally malnourished (grades II and III) remained so. It might be expected that with participation over a longer period of time the percentage of children failing to adjust to grade I and above would be still lower. Accordingly the basic runs of the simulation program assume $c_{12} = 0.1$ and $c_{13} = 0.15$.

UPPER AND LOWER BOUND COEFFICIENTS

The coefficients defining the upper and lower bounds of $L_{ia}(I,S)$ can be calculated by noting that at extreme values the lower bound of $L_{ia}(I,S)$ is α_{iaL} and the upper bound is $\alpha_{iau} + \alpha_{iaL}$. At the baseline lower limits for the morbidity rates (P^L), the morbidity function can be written

[a] The data are part of the NINCDS Collaborative Perinatal Project U.S. Department of Health, Education, and Welfare). We are grateful for the permission of Joseph Drage and Stanley Garn to use this data and for the research assistance of Karin Hoff in its analysis.

$$P_{ia}^{L} = a_{ia}\alpha_{iaL} + \sum b_{ija}P_{ja}^{L} + c_{ia}P_{ia-1}^{L},$$

which can be solved for α_{iaL} in terms of the baseline data (P^L) and the a, b, and c coefficients previously calculated,

$$\alpha_{iaL} = \frac{1}{a_{ia}} \left(P_{ia}^{L} - \sum b_{ija}P_{ja}^{L} - c_{ia}P_{ia-1}^{L}\right) \tag{5A-2}$$

Similarly, the upper bound coefficient can be calculated from

$$\alpha_{iaU} = \frac{1}{a_{ia}} \left(P_{ia}^{U} - \sum b_{ija}P_{ja}^{U} - c_{ia}P_{ia-1}^{U}\right) - \alpha_{iaL}$$

INTERVENTION IMPACT COEFFICIENTS

Two slightly different procedures are used to convert the survey responses to impact coefficients in the morbidity equations, depending on whether or not the response frame includes a consideration of the external effects of the intervention. For both procedures the same steps are involved in the conversion of the responses to impact coefficients. First, the responses are reinterpreted as partial derivatives giving the change in the morbidity rate with a change in an intervention. Second, the morbidity functions are differentiated partially with respect to each intervention. This results in an expression containing the baseline morbidity and intervention rates as well as the coefficient of unknown value. Third, the partial derivatives from the two sources—the survey responses and the morbidity equations—are set equal and solved for the unknown coefficient. Finally, the coefficient is calculated as a point estimate using the survey responses and baseline levels of the interventions and morbidity rates.

Calculation of the Impact Coefficients in the Case of no Externalities

Where there are no externalities, that is, where the indirect effects of the intervention are zero, the response, R_{iak}, gives the difference between the morbidity rate in a population without (wo) a given intervention (the kth) and a population with (w) the intervention,

$$R_{iak} = \frac{P_{ia}^{wk} - P_{ia}^{wok}}{P_{ia}^{wok}} \tag{5A-4}$$

which, if the intervention is an improvement, will be less than zero. The actual morbidity rate for the entire population is a weighted average of

P_{ia}^{wk} and P_{ia}^{wok} where the weight is the proportion (I_k) of the population covered by the intervention;

$$P_{ia} = I_k P_{ia}^{wk} + (1 - I_k) \cdot P_{ia}^{wok} \qquad \text{(5A–5)}$$

assuming no externalities (that is, P_{ia}^{wk} does not change with I_k) the change in the population morbidity rate with a change in the intervention is

$$\frac{\partial P_{ia}}{\partial I_k} = P_{ia}^{wk} - P_{ia}^{wok} \qquad \text{(5A–6)}$$

Solving equations (5A–4) and (5A–5) for P_{ia}^{wk} and P_{ia}^{wok} and, substituting in (5A–6) gives

$$\frac{\partial P_{ia}}{\partial I_k} = \frac{R_{iak} P_{ia}}{1 + R_{iak} \cdot I_k} \qquad \text{(5A–7)}$$

Turning to the morbidity function, equation (5A–1), the change in the morbidity rate with a change in the intervention is

$$\frac{\partial P_{ia}}{\partial I_k} = \alpha_{iak} \left(\frac{\alpha_{iaU} e^{-Z}}{(1 + e^{-Z})^2} \right) \cdot a_{ia} \qquad \text{(5A–8)}$$

Equating (5A–7) and (5A–8) and solving for the impact coefficient, α_{iak}, gives,

$$\alpha_{iak} = \left(\frac{R_{iak} P_{ia}}{1 + R_{iak} I_k} \right) \left(\frac{(1 + e^{-Z_{ia}})^2}{\alpha_{iaU} e^{-Z_{ia}}} \right) \cdot \frac{1}{a_{ia}} \qquad \text{(5A–9)}$$

A point estimate of α_{iak} is obtained at the baseline values of the morbidity and intervention rates (P^B, I^B) by noting that at the baseline point on the morbidity function

$$L^B = L_{ia}^B(I, S) = \frac{1}{a_{ia}} \left(P_{ia}^B - \sum b_{ija} P_{ja}^B - c_{ia} P_{ia-1} \right) \qquad \text{(5A–10)}$$

and

$$Z_{ia}^B = -\ln \left(\frac{\alpha_{iaU}}{L_{ia}^B - \alpha_{iaL}} - 1 \right) \qquad \text{(5A–11)}$$

Given the previously calculated values for the upper and lower bound coefficients (α_{iaU} and α_{iaL}) and the linear weight coefficients (a, b, c) a value of Z_{ia}^B can be computed. The impact coefficient is then calculated from equation (5A–9) using the baseline data, I_k^B, P_{ia}^B, Z_{ia}^B and the survey response R_{iak}.

Using the computed values of the α_{iak} coefficients, the constant in the Z

function, α_{iao}, can be chosen so that the baseline morbidity rate is reproduced by baseline values of the interventions.

$$\alpha_{iao} = Z^B_{ia} - \sum \alpha_{iak} I^B_k$$

Computation of the coefficients on the socioeconomic variables proceeds in the same manner as used for the intervention impact coefficients.

Impact Coefficients in the Case of Externalities

For some interventions survey respondents indicated that an improvement in an intervention would also decrease the incidence of disease in that part of the population already receiving an intervention as well as decreasing the morbidity rate in new recipients. In this case we distinguish between responses for a reference population with the intervention,

$$R^X_{iak} = \frac{P^{wk*}_{ia} - P^{wk}_{ia}}{P^{wk}_{ia}} \tag{5A–12}$$

and for a reference population not having the intervention,

$$R_{iak} = \frac{P^{wk*}_{ia} - P^{wok}_{ia}}{P^{wok}_{ia}} \tag{5A–13}$$

where P^{wk*}_{ia} is the new morbidity rate in the population having the intervention and P^{wk}_{ia} is the old morbidity rate for those with the intervention before the coverage of the intervention was increased. As in the previous section, the morbidity rate for the entire population before extension of the intervention is

$$P_{ia} = I_k P^{wk}_{ia} + (1 - I_k) \cdot P^{wok}_{ia}$$

In this case the change in the population morbidity rate with a change in the intervention is

$$\frac{\partial P_{ia}}{\partial I_k} = I_k \frac{\partial P^{wk}_{ia}}{\partial I_k} + P^{wk}_{ia} - P^{wok}_{ia}$$

assuming that externalities affecting that part of the population that continues to do without the intervention are negligible $(\partial P^{wok}_{ia} / \partial I_k = 0)$. We note, using (5A–12) that $\partial P^{wk}_{ia} / \partial I_k$ can be approximated by $(P^{wk*}_{ia} - P^{wk}_{ia}) / \Delta I_k = R^X_{iak} P^{wk}_{ia} / \Delta I_k$ so that, approximately,

$$\frac{\partial P_{ia}}{\partial I_k} = (I_k R^X \cdot P^{wk}_{ia} / \Delta I_k) + P^{wk}_{ia} - P^{wok}_{ia} \tag{5A–14}$$

Solving equations (5A–5), (5A–12), and (5A–13) for P_{ia}^{wk}, P_{ia}^{wok}, and P_{ia}^{wk*} and substituting in (5A–14) gives

$$\frac{\partial P_{ia}}{\partial I_k} = \frac{P_{ia}}{D}\left[\frac{I_k}{\Delta I}\cdot\frac{R^X}{(1+R^X)} + \frac{1}{1+R^X} - \frac{1}{1+R}\right] \qquad (5A\text{–}15)$$

$$D = \frac{I_k}{1+R_{iak}^X} + \frac{(1-I_k)}{1+R_{iak}}$$

Equating (5A–15) with the comparable partial derivative of the morbidity function (see equation 5A–8) and solving for the impact coefficient, α_{iak}, yields

$$\alpha_{iak} = \frac{P_{ia}T}{D}\left(\frac{(1+e^{-Z_{ia}})^2}{\alpha_{iaU}e^{-Z_{ia}}}\right)\cdot\frac{1}{a_{ia}} \qquad (5A\text{–}16)$$

where T is the expression in brackets on the right-hand side of equation (5A–15). A point estimate of α_{iak} can now be calculated using the baseline data, P^B, I^B, Z^B as computed in the previous section, ΔI as given in the survey questions ($\Delta I = 0.5$), and the survey responses, R_{iak}^X and R_{iak}.

CONSISTENCY AMONG BASE LINE DATA AND *a*, *b*, *c* COEFFICIENTS

In order to calculate Z^B (see equation 5A–11) it is necessary that

$$Y = \frac{\alpha_{iaU}}{L_{ia}^B - \alpha_{iaL}} > 1 \qquad (5A\text{–}17)$$

This requirement can be translated into a restriction on the relationship among the baseline data by substituting equations (5A–2), (5A–3), and (5A–10) in (5A–17). This gives

$$Y = \frac{P_{ia}^U - P_{ia}^L - \sum b_{ija}P_{ja}(P_{ja}^U - P_{ja}^L) - c_{ia}(P_{ia-1}^U - P_{ia-1}^L)}{P_{ia}^B - P_{ia}^L - \sum b_{ija}P_{ja}(P_{ja}^B - P_{ja}^L) - c_{ia}(P_{ia-1}^U - P_{ia-1}^L)}$$

which must be greater than one if the baseline data and *a*, *b*, *c* coefficients are to be mutually consistent.

NOTE

1. See Joe D. Wray, "Direct Nutrition Intervention and the Control of Diarrheal Diseases in Pre-School Children," mimeographed, n.d.

Appendix 5B

Specification of the Coefficients in the Usage Functions

The usage coefficients are based on the responses summarized in Table 5–6. The method of calculation of the usage coefficients is slightly different from the method used for the morbidity coefficients because the survey questions for usage asked for absolute levels relating to given levels of the intervention and socioeconomic variables rather than asking for changes directly. Differentiating the usage equation with respect to the socioeconomic (SES) variables and imputing a comparable change in usage with a change in each SES variable from the survey response produces an estimate of the SES coefficients. The constant in the logit equation is then chosen so that the function passes through the baseline usage rate. Finally, using the SES coefficients and constant, the intervention coefficients are calculated to reproduce the absolute usage levels provided by the survey responses.

Given the usage equation,

$$u_{la} = \frac{1}{1 + e^{-U_{la}}} \tag{5B–1}$$

where $U_{la} = \gamma_{lao} + \sum \gamma_{lak} I_k + \sum \gamma_{las} S_s$, the change in usage with a change in a socioeconomic variable is

$$\frac{\partial u_{la}}{\partial s_s} = u_{la}(1 - u_{la}) \cdot \gamma_{las}$$

or, solving for the unknown coefficient,

$$\gamma_{las} = \frac{\partial u}{\partial s} \cdot \left[\frac{1}{u_{la}(1 - u_{la})} \right] \tag{5B–2}$$

From the responses, we know the level of usage at the baseline, u_{la}^{B}, and with a doubling of the socioeconomic variable, u_{la}^{s}. This allows an approximation of $\partial u / \partial s$ to be calculated as $(u_{la}^{s} - u_{l}^{B})/S_{s}^{B}$, which may be substituted in (5B–2) to give an estimate of γ_{las} in terms of the response u_{la}^{s} and baseline data.

$$\gamma_{las} = \left[\frac{u_{l}^{s} - u_{l}^{B}}{S_{s}^{B}} \right] \left[\frac{1}{u_{la}^{B}(1 - u_{la}^{B})} \right] \tag{5B–3}$$

Because the baseline level of the interventions affecting usage is zero (at the baseline date there were no mass media or promotora programs), a point estimate of the constant γ_{lao} can be calculated using the estimates of γ_{las} given by equation (5B–3), so that the usage equation reproduces the baseline rate at the baseline values of the SES variables,

$$\gamma_{lao} = -\ln \left[\frac{1}{u_{la}^{B}} - 1 \right] - \sum \gamma_{las} S_{s}^{B} \tag{5B–4}$$

Finally, point estimates[a] of the intervention coefficients can be calculated from the survey responses, u_{la}^{k}, and baseline data,

$$\gamma_{lak} = -\ln \left[\frac{1}{u_{la}^{k}} - 1 \right] - \gamma_{lao} - \sum \gamma_{las} S_{s}^{B} \tag{5B–5}$$

[a] Estimates of the intervention coefficients could also be made using the same procedure as for the SES coefficients, but the point estimate in equation (5B–5) is a more accurate procedure and was made possible by the fact that the responses give the change in usage as the coverage of the intervention goes from zero to 100 percent.

Chapter 6

Resource Requirements, Resource Availability, and Demographic Constraints

INTRODUCTION

Differences in costs are perhaps the most important reason that specific quantitative results and policy conclusions obtained from an application of the resource allocation model in one region or country can not be transferred or, at least, immediately applied in another region. The costs of the activities considered are greatly affected by the mode of delivery, the organization of health institutions, the availability of related technology, and the state of local resource markets, and all of these things vary greatly among regions. In deriving the resource costs for the hypothetical community modeled here, we have worked with local budgets and taken institutions, technology, and prices from the five *barrios* in Cali, Colombia, described earlier in Chapter 4. This was possible because there are prototypical programs, of the type being considered as potential health activities in this study, currently being carried out in the Cali area with the assistance of the Colombian or local governments, the Ford Foundation, USAID, the PRIMOPS project, and others.[a]

We have identified as potential resource constraints (1) total costs; (2) total supplies costs; (3) physician time; (4) registered nurse time;

[a] Information about the resource use and operation of these programs was obtained through the cooperation of program administrators. We are especially grateful for the help of Dr. Bernardo Correa who supplied immunization costs and Dr. Jaime Rodriguez who provided information related to PRIMOPS programs.

(5) auxiliary nurse time; (6) bed days available; and (7) capacity of physical facilities. Total monetary costs include expenditures for administration, salaries of personnel, depreciation on capital equipment and buildings, and supplies. The costs of supplies and expendable equipment are also analyzed separately because budget items in this category can be regarded by administrators as more easily changed over a planning period than are the other items in total costs, such as salaries and depreciation, that are apt to entail longer-run budget committments. Physician time includes administrative as well as service uses of time. The same is true of registered nurse time (which, for most of the programs considered, is almost entirely administrative time) and to some extent auxiliary nurse time. Both bed days and physical capacity represent the use of physical facilities but a distinction is made between bed capacity, which is primarily a constraint on the number of inpatients, and the use of other forms of physical capital.[b] Inpatient and outpatient care for children, examinations and treatment of women, institutional deliveries, and visits to the well-baby clinic all make use of health center and hospital physical facilities apart from bed capacity. Physical capacity is measured in monetary units only as a convenience and could, conceptually, have been measured in other units such as square meters.

For most of the activities the costs are obtained by dividing total budget figures by numbers of units of services delivered over the budget period. This represents a notably different approach as compared to building up costs from time and motion studies of the separate job components comprising the activities.[1] Budget analysis is a more practical approach because it relies on available information and data normally gathered as part of administrative operations. The use of budget information also has the advantage of including preparation, administration, and normal slack time or changes in pace that might be omitted by timing specific operations. Budget analysis does have the disadvantage of making it difficult to cost separate interventions that are included together in an aggregate budget. A number of assumptions have been used below to allow the disaggregation of the budgets. An effort has been made to outline the assumptions. It was felt that the resource costs obtained were sufficiently accurate for the broad comparisons of cost effectiveness to be made in the child mortality project; but, because of the necessary assumptions and because in some cases the number of units of services delivered were not directly recorded and instead estimates were made by program administrators, the unit costs given below should not be used for other purposes outside of the context of the present project. Table 6–14 summarizes the resource costs per unit of activity. The derivation of the unit costs is discussed in the section that follows. Costs are based on 1977–1978 prices and wages.

[b] The allocation of physical capacity should not be confused with depreciation, which represents the cost of replacing capial equipment and buildings used over the planning period and that is included in total costs.

RESOURCE COSTS

Promotora

Promotora costs include the direct and supervisory costs of service delivery and the depreciated cost of training. The first four columns of Table 6–1 present the costs per visit assuming 264 visits per month per promotora, salaries as given in Table 6–2, and an eight-week training program that uses 132 physician hours and 704 registered nurse hours to train thirty promotoras. To the extent that 264 visits per month is an optimistic figure, costs are underestimated. In the PRIMOPS program, used as the basis for the calculations, the rate of personnel turnover is low and the rate of depreciation of training through attrition is estimated to be only 0.07 per year. This contrasts markedly with the rates observed in rural areas, where migration of trained health promotoras is an important factor. For this reason, although training is not a large component of resource use in the promotora program in Cali, it may be a significant factor in other regions. The negligible use of medical doctor time is attributable to the fact that all administration, both in training and delivery, is carried out by registered nurses. Physician time (a total of 264 minutes per promotora trained) is used only for teaching. For a promotora program involving three visits per year, the costs per family for a twenty-eight-day period are given in the last column of Table 6–1.

Several other activities involve the promotora either directly or indirectly. An unattended home delivery followed by a promotora visit has the costs given in column 4 of Table 6–1. The costs of promotora services in the delivery of immunizations are incorporated directly in the costs of the immunization activities. In other cases where the promotora is involved in

Table 6–1. Promotora Costs per Visit.

	Per Visit				
	Service Delivery				*Per 28 Days per Family*
Resource Category	*Direct (Col. 1)*	*Supervisory (Col. 2)*	*Training (Col. 3)*	*Total (Col. 4)*	*(Col. 5)*
Total budget (pesos)	18.182	3.685	.209	22.076	5.081
Supplies budget (pesos)	3.031		.005	3.036	.699
Medical doctor (minutes)			.006	.006	.001
Reg. nurse (minutes)	1.846		.031	1.877	.432
Aux. nurse (minutes)	4.000			4.000	.921
Capital capacity[a] (pesos)	—	—	—	4.200	.969

[a] Not calculated by separate components.

Table 6–2. Personnel Salaries (Colombian pesos per four weeks).

Staff	Salary
Promotora	4,000
Auxiliary nurse	5,039
Registered nurse	10,160
Medical doctor	16,500
Midwife	4,500

the delivery of an activity, the role of the promotora is modeled by an appropriate restriction on the choice of activities in the computer program. Thus, the supplemental iron for all women is delivered by the promotora and restricted to be less than or equal to the coverage of the promotora. Also, nutritional programs for children involve screening and preliminary identification by the promotora and the coverage of nutritional programs is restricted to be less than or equal to the coverage by the promotora activity.

Midwife Delivery

Table 6–3 summarizes the costs of a midwife delivery, breaking down the total costs into training and the direct cost of the service. The costs were calculated under the assumptions that midwife training depreciates at a rate of 0.2, reflecting the higher rate of turnover among midwives as compared to promotoras, and that a six-week training program for eighteen midwives will involve seven and one-half weeks of registered nurse time. The program as organized in the PRIMOPS area does not use physicians either for training or supervision, but does make relatively heavy use of registered nurse and auxiliary nurse time. The unit costs are calculated per delivery and assume one delivery per day and twenty working days per twenty-eight-day period.

Outpatient Care and Well-Baby Clinic

The costs of outpatient visits are calculated in terms of a "standard" or "unit" visit requiring fiteen minutes of direct auxiliary nurse time. The proportional use of time for various types of visits was expressed in terms of

Table 6–3. Midwife Costs per Delivery

Resource Category	Direct Costs	Training	Total
Total budget (pesos)	259.241	.882	260.123
Supplies budget (pesos)	4.167		4.168
Reg. nurse (minutes)	1.500	.917	2.417
Aux. nurse (minutes)	60.000		60.000

Table 6–4. Outpatient Care Factors (expressed in terms of a standard visit).

Purpose	*Factor*	*Unit*
Standard	1.0	visit
Exam of neonatal child	1.0	one exam
Outpatient care of 1–12 month child[a]	1.6	per illness
Outpatient care of 12–60 month child[a]	1.6	per illness
Well-baby clinic 1–12[b]	1.33	per child of 1–12 months covered by the program
Well-baby clinic 12–60[c]	2.00	per child of 12–60 months covered by the program

[a] Assumes that 60 percent of patients in this age group who receive curative care return for a second visit.
[b] Assumes two visits with a length of two-thirds of a standard visit.
[c] Assumes three visits with a length of two-thirds of a standard visit.

the standard visit and multiplied by the total number of visits of particular types to get a total number of standard unit visit equivalents.[2] Budgeted resources in the various categories were then divided by this figure to get the resource use per standard visit. Finally an outpatient care factor that represents the relative use of health center services for various purposes was calculated. The factor represents the length of the type of visit times the number of visits involved for each purpose. Table 6–4 gives the factors

Table 6–5. Outpatient Clinic Resource Use.

Resource	*(1) Use per Standard Visit Unit*	*(2) Use per Illness for 1–12 and 12–60 Age Groups*[a]	*(3) Use per Child Covered by the Well-Baby Clinic per 28 Days*[b]	
			0–12	*12–60*
Total budget (pesos)	84.424	135.078	9.357	3.238
Supplies budget (pesos)	6.170	9.872	.684	.236
Medical doctor (minutes)	5.942	9.507	.659	.228
Reg. nurse (minutes)	7.444	11.904	.825	.286
Aux. nurse (minutes)	31.509	50.414	3.492	1.209
Capital capacity (pesos)	15.937	25.499	1.766	.611

[a] Column 2 = column 1 times the outpatient care factor in Table 6–4.
[b] This column represents the resource cost for a standard visit multiplied by the appropriate outpatient care factor in Table 6–4, divided by the total number of 28-day periods in the relevant age group.

representing the relative use of health center outpatient care facilities for various types of visits. Column 1 of Table 6–5 gives the cost of a standard visit and represents an average of the costs of care in the Antonio Narino health center and the Carlos Carmona outpatient facility. Because the data are derived from budget totals, they include the cost of backup outpatient clinical facilities, overhead, and personnel time not directly involved in the visit.

Inpatient Care

The available budget data were not sufficiently disaggregated to distinguish cost differences per bed day for the three age groups. Assuming that the costs are approximately the same per bed day for each age group, Column 1 of Table 6–6 gives a weighted average of resource costs for inpatient care in the university and Carlos Carmona hospitals. The weights are derived from the assumption that 0.82 of inpatients in the five-*barrio* area will use the Carlos Carmona facility while the remaining 0.18 will use the university hospital. Columns 2, 3, and 4 represent the resource use per illness and represent column 1 multiplied by the average number of bed days for each age category. The data did not allow a distinction of length of stay by morbidity classification. The average length of stay is assumed to be four days for the 0–1 age group, three and a half days for the 1–12, and three days for the 12–60. These data are approximated using records for the average number of days per discharge from Carlos Carmona Hospital.

Institutional Delivery

The costs of a health system delivery represents the weighted average of costs of inpatient obstetric care in the university and the Carlos Carmona

Table 6–6. Resource Use for Inpatient Care and Institutional Delivery.

		Use per Average Illness			
Resource Category	*Use per Bed Day (Col. 1)*	*0–1 (Col. 2)*	*1–12 (Col. 3)*	*12–60 (Col. 4)*	*Use per Delivery (Col. 5)*
Total budget (pesos)	1010.811	4043.244	3537.835	3032.430	2049.134
Supplies budget (pesos)	419.160	1676.640	1467.060	1257.480	758.478
Medical doctor (minutes)	64.414	257.656	255.449	193.242	142.200
Reg. nurse (minutes)	16.921	67.684	59.224	50.763	40.350
Aux. nurse (minutes)	187.612	750.448	656.642	562.836	516.840
Bed days	1.000	4.000	3.500	3.000	2.150
Capital capacity (pesos)	3341.910	13367.620	11696.670	10025.720	6461.000

Table 6–7. Resource Use for Annual Examinations of Women of Childbearing Age.

Resource	Health Center (One Visit per Year)	Promotora (0.2 of a "Normal" Visit)	Laboratory Tests[a] (0.5 of All Exams)	Additional Supervision of Promotora	Total per Year per Woman	Total per 28 Days per Woman
Total budget (pesos)	84.424	13.246	18.000		115.670	8.898
Supplies budget (pesos)	6.170	1.824	18.000		25.995	2.000
Medical doctor (minutes)	5.942	.004			5.946	.457
Reg. nurse (minutes)	7.444	1.126		1.500	10.071	.775
Aux. nurse (minutes)	31.509	2.400			33.909	2.608
Capital capacity (pesos)	15.937				15.937	1.226

[a] The cost of a test for urinary tract infection is 26 pesos and the cost of a hemoglobin test is 10 pesos making a total cost of 36 pesos for both tests. In practice, the tests are given to 50 percent of women having an examination.

Table 6–8. Costs of Treatments for Women of Childbearing Age.

	Cost per Treatment		*Cost per 28 Days per Woman Requiring Treatment after Annual Examination*	
Resource	*Infection (Col. 1)*	*Anemia (Col. 2)*	*Infection (Col. 3)*	*Anemia (Col. 4)*
Total budget (pesos)	834.424	115.424	64.011	8.854
Supplies budget (pesos)	756.170	37.170	58.008	2.851
Medical doctor (minutes)	5.942	5.942	.456	.456
Reg. nurse (minutes)	7.444	7.444	.571	.571
Aux. nurse (minutes)	31.509	31.509	2.417	2.417
Capital capacity (pesos)	15.937	15.937	1.223	1.223

hospitals and of obstetrical services provided by the Antonio Narino health center. The weights are 0.1, 0.45, and 0.45, respectively, and represent the proportion of all institutional deliveries in the five-*barrio* area using the services of each of the three alternative facilities. The costs are given in column 5 of Table 6–6.

Examinations and Treatment of Women of Childbearing Age

Motivation and enrollment of eligible women require additional promotora time equal to one-fifth of the normal promotora visit per woman per year. An annual examination is given to each woman and laboratory tests for infection and hemoglobin are conducted in the 50 percent of the examinations where sufficient symptoms are present. Table 6–7 presents a breakdown of the resources required by the examination. Column 5 is the total cost per woman for the annual examination and column 6 is the cost per twenty-eight days per woman covered by the program.

The cost of treatments for infection and anemia are given in Table 6–8. The total costs include an additional health center control visit and additional supplies. The costs per twenty-eight days, given in columns 3 and 4, are based on the assumption that infected or anemic women require only one course of treatment over a one-year period. The cost of the treatment for infection is attributable to the relatively high cost of the necessary antibiotics. In contrast the supplies cost for the treatment of iron deficiency is low. As an alternative to the selective treatment of only iron-deficient women, a program covering all women entails the distribution by the promotora of an iron supplement. Although the direct costs of this program are low (7.154 pesos per twenty-eight days), since it does not require a health center visit, the coverage of the program is restricted to be less than or equal to the coverage of the promotora.

Examinations and Treatment of Pregnant Women

This activity consists of one health center visit of standard length for each suspected pregnancy. Because there are approximately 1.26 suspected pregnancies per actual pregnancy, the initial examination and detection requires 1.26 visit units per pregnancy. The initial examination is followed by control visits equal to one visit unit making a total of 2.26 visit units per pregnancy. Additional laboratory costs for the initial examination are 36 pesos per pregnancy. The total costs per pregnant woman examined are given in column 1 of Table 6–9. The cost of treating women who are found to have infections represents two additional control visits to the health center and the cost of antibiotics. The total cost per infected woman treated is given in column 2. Column 3 gives the cost of hygienic education of pregnant women in the health center. The cost represents the use of additional health center resources in lectures of one hour duration given to groups of eight women by an auxiliary nurse.

Other activities related to prenatal examinations are nutritional supplements for all pregnant women or women with high risk of low birth weight and the institutional delivery of high low-birth-weight- and birth-trauma-risk women. For these activities the examination is used for screening or enrollment. Although these activities do not require significant additional resources during the examination, the activities cannot occur without an examination, and the number of women covered is restricted to be less than or equal to the number of women covered by the prenatal examination.

Immunizations

Immunizations can be delivered through several channels: Promotora, well-baby clinics, at the time of examinations of pregnant women, or through special programs. The cost data used here relate to an ongoing

Table 6–9. Resource Costs of Prenatal Examinations and Treatments.

	Program Costs per Pregnancy		
Resource	*Examination*	*Treatment*	*Health Center Education*
Total budget (pesos)	226.798	918.848	42.212
Supplies budget (pesos)	49.948	762.340	3.085
Medical doctor (minutes)	13.429	11.884	2.971
Reg. nurse (minutes)	16.824	14.889	3.722
Aux. nurse (minutes)	71.210	63.018	15.755
Capital capacity (pesos)	36.092	31.940	7.969

Table 6–10. Resource Costs of Immunizations.

Resource	Tetanus (Pregnant Women)	DPT & Polio	Measles	Total: DPT, Polio, Measles
Total budget (pesos)	42.399	159.192	40.936	200.128
Supplies budget (pesos)	10.364	31.051	24.920	55.971
Medical doctor (minutes)	.012	2.995	.375	3.370
Reg. nurse (minutes)	.098	23.496	2.937	26.433

program in Cali. The program is actually carried out in conjunction with services provided as part of the PRIMOPS project, and inoculations are delivered both by promotoras and in the health center. The costs presented in Table 6–10 represent the costs of the immunization including the cost of delivery by promotora. The costs are for a completed series of inoculations and assume two inoculations of pregnant women for tetanus, four shots for DPT plus polio, and one shot for measles.

Water and Sanitation

These costs represent the annualized capital costs of installation and connection for the activities under consideration and the cost of water supply for flush toilets and water sources. For home water supply it is assumed that the installation has a twenty-year life, that water costs 3.5 pesos per cubic meter, and that the average family (5.6 persons) would use 218 liters per day for nontoilet uses. For public water, it is assumed that the installation has a twenty-year life and would cover eight families and that the average family covered would use 8.4 liters per day. It is assumed that the latrine has a life of ten years, that the toilet installation has a life of fifteen years, and the sewage system a life of thirty years. The toilet is assumed to require 392 liters of water per family per day. The costs per twenty-eight days per family are summarized in Table 6–11.

Table 6–11. Water and Sanitation Resource Costs (per household).

	Water Supply		Sanitation	
Resource	Home	Public Spigot	Toilet	Latrine
Total budget (pesos)	76.711	15.146	109.878	6.786
Supplies budget (pesos)	21.403	8.232	38.416	

Table 6–12. Nutritional Program Resource Costs.

Resource	*Programs for Women, per Participant per 28 Days*	*Programs for Children, per Participant per 28 Days*
Total budget (pesos)	218.000	122.000
Supplies budget (pesos)	188.000	92.000
Aux. nurse (minutes)	62.870	62.870

Nutritional Programs

Table 6–12 gives the cost of the nutritional programs. Total costs include both nutritional supplies and the time of an auxiliary nurse who is involved with administration, motivation, and evaluation tasks related to the programs. The data represent the cost of an ongoing nutritional program in the Cali area. The program costs are assumed to be the same for all three of the programs affecting women and for the two programs for children. Costs given in the table are per participant. The design of the program includes screening the children for risk of malnutrition. In practice, 40 percent of all children covered by the program participate; costs per child covered by the program are therefore 40 percent of the values given in the table.

Mass Media

The cost of a comprehensive mass media program that uses radio, posters, billboards, and leaflets and that covers diarrhea, sanitation, breast feeding, and early detection of pregnancy is 200,000 pesos for a community of 10,000. The program is designed by the central government and does not require the time of local medical personnel. The cost of the program for the five-*barrio* area would be 8.438 pesos per family per twenty-eight days.

RESOURCE AVAILABILITY

The resource constraints for the hypothetical community are estimated by aggregating the budgets, staff time, and capital capacity for various health programs serving the five-*barrio* population in 1978. Table 6–13 gives the full budget for the promotora and immunization programs. The resources available from the health center and hospitals represent the proportional part of the total resources that is used by the study area and that applies to women and children in the age groups included in the

Table 6–13. Resources Available per 28 days[a]

Program Source	*Total Peso Budget* R_1	*Supplies Budget (Pesos)* R_2	*Physician Time (Minutes)* R_3	*Registered Nurse Time (Minutes)* R_4	*Auxiliary Nurse Time (Minutes)* R_5	*Bed Days* R_6	*Capital (Physical Capacity) (Pesos)* R_7
Promotora	69,738	9,590	19	5,929	12,636		173,600
Health center	100,769	7,364	9,216	3,379	60,826		247,296
Carlos Carmona	434,044	119,935	21,389	5,414	61,901	344	15,360,000
University hospital	700,061	398,816	72,192	19,852	211,661	463	19,468,800
Immunizations	48,842	14,311	808	6,332			
Nutrition[b]	305,000	230,000			157,175		
Water[b]	383,500	107,015					
Sanitation[b]	549,390	192,080					
Total	2,591,344	1,079,111	103,624	40,906	504,199	807	35,249,696
Total/Family	210.35	87.60	8.41	3.32	40.93	.07	2,861.41

[a] Resources for programs affecting women fifteen to forty-five years of age and children less than five.
[b] Resources needed to provide an arbitrary 0.25 of children with a nutritional program and 0.5 of all families with water and sanitation services.

analysis. Only the service time of medical personnel in the university hospital is included; teaching time is excluded. Nevertheless, the large number of interns and residents may inflate the estimated availability of physician time. The proportions of resources for the Antonio Narino Health Center, Carlos Carmona Hospital, and the university hospital that are allocated to women between fifteen and forty-five and to children less than five is estimated to be 0.64. It is also estimated that area residents constitute 100 percent of the total use of the Antonio Narino Health Center, 80 percent of the total use of Carlos Carmona, and 6 percent of the total use of the university hospital. Bed days available are calculated with the assumption that under normal operations, Carlos Carmona will have an 80 percent occupancy rate and the university hospital will have an 85 percent occupancy rate. Resources entered under the nutrition program are an estimate of the resources needed to provide an arbitrary 25 percent of children with the nutrition program. Resources entered under water and sanitary categories are sufficient to provide 50 percent of all families with public water and latrines. Although there may be other government programs and private expenditures providing some health resources, the items in the table constitute the preponderance of total resource availability. All data are given in terms of a twenty-eight-day period. The total amount of resources available per four-week period is given in the next to the last row of the table. These amounts serve as the reference level, R, for the resource constraints in the allocation experiments. The total amounts of resources per capita are given in the last row of the table. Because there are a number of special programs in the Cali area that would not be available to the hypothetical community being modeled, the optimizations in Chapter 8 are carried out using an arbitrary 75 percent of the resources given in Table 6–13 for the basic optimization experiment.[c]

RESOURCE CONSTRAINTS

Table 6–14 summarizes the resource requirements. The table gives the requirement, r_{ij}, of resource j per unit of activity X_i. A subsection (BOUND) of the simulation model contains the resource constraints that restrict the total use of each of the seven resources by all activities to be less than or equal to the total resource availability,

$$\sum_{i=1}^{32} r_{ij} X_i \leq R_j^* \qquad j = 1 \ldots 7$$

[c]That is, the reference level of resources in the Cali community is R and the hypothetical community is assumed to have only $0.75R$ available.

Table 6–14. Resource Requirements per Unit of Activity.

Activity (Abbrev.)	Sub-script X_i/R_i	Total Unit Costs (Pesos) 1	Supplies Costs (Pesos) 2	Physician Time (Minutes) 3	Registered Nurse Time (Minutes) 4	Auxiliary Nurse Time (Minutes) 5	Bed Days 6	Use of Capital (Physical Capacity) (Pesos) 7	Unit[a]
PROMOTER	1	5.081	.698	.002	.432	.921	.000	12.682	per family/mo.
AWEXAM	2	8.898	2.000	.457	.775	2.608	.000	1.227	per eligible women/mo.
PWEXAM	3	226.798	49.945	13.429	16.824	71.210	—	36.092	per exam
AWTXINF	4	834.424	756.170	5.942	7.444	31.509	—	15.937	per treatment
AWTXAN	5	7.154	7.154	—	—	—	—	0.000	per participant/mo.
AFEDEFTX	6	115.424	37.170	5.942	7.444	31.509	—	15.937	per treatment
PWTXINF	7	918.848	762.340	11.884	14.888	63.018	—	31.940	per treatment
PWNUTLBW	8	218.000	188.000	—	—	62.870	—	—	per participant/mo.
PWTETIMM	9	42.399	10.364	.012	.098	—	—	—	per visit
PWHCED	10	42.212	3.085	2.971	3.722	15.755	—	7.969	per visit
PWNUT	11	218.000	188.000	—	—	62.870	—	—	per participant/mo.
DELIN	12	2049.130	758.480	142.200	40.350	516.840	2.150	6461.000	per delivery
DEL MW	13	260.123	4.167	—	2.417	60.000	—	—	per delivery
DEL&PROM	14	22.076	3.056	.006	1.877	4.000	—	54.954	per delivery
DELINLBW	15	2049.130	758.480	142.200	40.350	516.840	2.150	6461.000	per delivery
1 OUTP	16	84.424	6.170	5.942	7.444	31.509	—	15.937	per illness
1 INP	17	4043.244	1676.640	257.656	67.684	750.448	4.000	13367.620	per illness
H2O HOME	18	76.711	21.403	—	—	—	—	—	per family/mo.
H2O WALK	19	15.146	8.232	—	—	—	—	—	per family/mo.
TOILET	20	109.878	38.416	—	—	—	—	—	per family/mo.
LATRINE	21	6.786	—	—	—	—	—	—	per family/mo.
MMEDIA	22	8.438	8.438	—	—	—	—	—	per family/mo.

Table 6–14. *(Continued)*

Activity (Abbrev.)	*Sub-script* X_i/R_i	*Total Unit Costs (Pesos)* 1	*Supplies Costs (Pesos)* 2	*Physician Time (Minutes)* 3	*Registered Nurse Time (Minutes)* 4	*Auxiliary Nurse Time (Minutes)* 5	*Bed Days* 6	*Use of Capital (Physical Capacity) (Pesos)* 7	*Unit*[a]
IMMDPTPM	23	200.128	55.971	3.370	26.433	—	—	—	per immunized child
2 WBC	24	9.357	.684	.659	.825	3.492	—	1.766	per participant/mo.
2 NUTCH	25	48.800	36.800	—	—	25.148	—	—	per child/mo.
2 NUTBF	26	218.000	188.000	—	—	62.870	—	—	per participant/mo.
2 OUTP	27	48.800	36.800	9.507	11.904	50.414	—	25.499	per illness
2 INP	28	3537.835	1467.835	225.449	59.224	656.642	3.500	11696.670	per illness
3 WBC	29	3.238	.236	.228	.286	1.209	—	.611	per participant/mo.
3 NUTCH	30	48.800	36.800	—	—	25.148	—	—	per child/mo.
3 OUTP	31	135.078	9.872	9.507	11.904	50.414	—	25.499	per illness
3 INP	32	3032.430	1257.480	193.242	50.763	562.836	3.000	10025.720	per illness

[a] One unit month = twenty-eight days.

In the optimization experiments, several different levels of resources, all fractional multiples of the resource levels given at the bottom of Table 6–13, are used for R_j^* in order to examine differences in the optimum activity levels under alternative degrees of resource scarcity.

EPIDEMIOLOGICAL AND DEMOGRAPHIC CONSTRAINTS

All activities are also constrained by the size of epidemiological and demographic groups. Resources would, of course, be wasted if the scale of activities were allowed to be greater than the potential target

Table 6–15. Epidemiological and Population Constraints.

Description of Constraint[a]	*Subscript (N_i)*	*Value*	*Comment*
Families[b]	1	12319	
Women aged 15–19 years[b]	2	15412	
Pregnancies/month	3	266	Assumes a crude birth rate of 0.045 per year and 10 percent aborted or dead on arrival[c]
Infected women/month	4	119	Estimated 10 percent infection rate[d]
Anemic women/month	5	59	Estimated 5 percent anemic rate[d]
Infected pregnant women/month	6	27	Estimated 10 percent infection rate[d]
LBW risk pregnancies/month	7	69	Estimated 26 percent rate[e]
Births/month	8	239	Assumes a crude birth rate of 0.045 per year[e]
LBWW and BT risk births/month	9	61	Estimated 26 percent rate[e]

[a] One unit month = twenty-eight days.

[b] Patrick Marnane, "Primops Background Information, Community Profile of the U.V.P. Area" (mimeograph, Tulane University, School of Public Health, August 1975).

[c] The birth rate is based on a model life table approximating this population. The proportion of pregnancies terminating as abortions or still born children is based on a table in Jaime Rodriquez and Jesus Rico, eds., *Componentes Evaluativos de la Atencion Primeria*, Programa de la Investigacion en Modelos de Prestacion de Servicios de Salud (PRIMOPS), Cali, Colombia, 1978.

[d] Unpublished estimates by PRIMOPS personnel. The infection estimates are approximately consistent with data in Alfonso Santemaria and Luis Daza, *Investigacion de Riesgo Materno—Infantil*, Programa PRIMOPS, Ministerio de Salud, Colombia, 1978. The estimate of anemia is higher than the Santemaria/Daza estimate but was felt to be a closer approximation to the correct rate.

[e] High-risk pregnancies have been defined as those in which three or more risk factors, such as hypertension or anemia of the mother, maternal size less than 150 centimeters or maternal weight less than 40 kilograms, and infections are present. The estimate is based on the analysis of Santemaria and Daza cited above.

Table 6–16. Relationship Between Demographic Constraints and Activities

Activity		Applicable Demographic Constraint	Activity		Applicable Demographic Constraint
Description	*Subscript* (X_i)	*(Subscript)* (N_k)	*Description*	*Subscript* (X_i)	*(Subscript)* (N_k)
PROMOTER	1	1	1INP	17	8
AWEXAM	2	2	H2O HOME	18	1
PWEXAM	3	3	H2O WALK	19	1
AWTXINF	4	4	TOILET	20	1
AWTXAN	5	2	LATRINE	21	1
AFEDEFTX	6	5	MMEDIA	22	1
PWTXINF	7	6	IMMDPTPM	23	[a]
PWNUTLBW	8	7	2WBC	24	[a]
PWTETIMM	9	3	2NUTCH	25	[a]
PWHCED	10	3	2NUTBF	26	[a]
PWNUT	11	3	2OUTP	27	[a]
DELIN	12	8	2INP	28	[a]
DELMW	13	8	3WBC	29	[a]
DEL&PROM	14	8	3NUTCH	30	[a]
DELINLBW	15	9	3OUTP	31	[a]
1OUTP	16	8	3INP	32	[a]

[a] The constraining population is not known prior to computation of the number of survivors from one age group to the next. As a practical means of placing an initial upper bound on the search for optimum activity levels, these activities are given artificial constraints calculated from the number of births, N_8, and assuming total survival. The actual size of the demographic group varies with the success of earlier health activities and is obtained after the number of survivors is calculated for earlier age groups.

populations. For example, the total number of households covered by the promotora cannot be greater than the number of households in the modeled community. Tables 6–15 and 6–16 summarize the population constraints. Table 6–16 gives the applicable demographic constraint, N_k, for each activity;

$$X_i \leq N_k \qquad i = 1 \ldots 32 \qquad k = f(i)$$

The specific values for N_k are given in Table 6–15. The epidemiological constraints are conveniently incorporated in the optimization program as absolute limits on the search for optimum activity levels and are not included in BOUND.

Epidemiological and demographic constraints also enter the model as denominators in the calculation of the proportional coverage of the activities,

$$x_i = X_i / N_k \qquad i = 1 \ldots 32 \qquad k = f(i)$$

where k is given from Table 6–15. In the calculation of the per capita level of activities for age groups 2 and 3 the actual size of the demographic group varies with the success of earlier health activities and is obtained within the computer program after the number of survivors for earlier age groups is computed.

ADDITIONAL RESTRICTIONS

In addition to the resource and demographic constraints, there are also a number of restrictions on the relationships between activities. These constraints restrict (1) the sum of institutional deliveries, midwife deliveries, and unattended deliveries followed by promotora to be less than or equal to the total number of births; (2) the total of home and public water to be less than or equal to the number of households; (3) the total of latrine and toilet activities to be less than the number of households; and (4) the total of inpatient and outpatient care to be less than or equal to the number of cases requiring treatment. Other restrictions require that the proportional coverage of treatments for pregnant women and all women be less than the proportional coverage of examinations for each group, and that the proportional coverage of nutritional programs for children and the iron program for women be less than the proportional coverage of households by the promotora. In all there are sixteen additional restrictions of this type. The precise formulation of the restrictions is given in lines 23–39 of the computer subprogram BOUND in the Appendix. These restrictions reflect the organization of programs in the hypothetical community and, of course, might change considerably in a reformulation of the model to fit other specific communities.

SUMMARY

This chapter discusses the resource use, resource availability, demographic constraints, and institutional restrictions that restrain the scale of health activities affecting children in the model community. The data are obtained for a community in Cali, Colombia. In terms of peso cost per unit the most expensive activities are inpatient care, institutional deliveries, and treatment for infection. These activities also have the greatest unit use of personnel time. The least expensive activities per unit are health promotion, latrines, well-baby clinics, and iron supplements.

The total costs for a given activity are also related to the size of the demographic target group as well as the unit costs. For instance, nutritional programs and immunizations for all children have high total costs relative to, say, midwife delivery; although the unit costs are of roughly the same magnitude, there is a tenfold difference in the size of the demographic base. Thus, the demographic constraints as well as the resource constraints play an important role in determining the optimum scale of activities.

Intervention impacts and resource costs are equally important in determining the most cost-effective allocation of resources. Both of these aspects of the model may vary from one community to another but the variation in costs would be expected to be far greater than the variation in impacts of identical programs. Cost differentials between communities are an important reason that the optimal allocation for one community—for instance, the hypothetical community modeled in this study—may not be extendable to other communities with different institutional and demographic conditions.

NOTES

1. The time and motion approach to unit costs was used by Martin Feldstein, M. A. Piot, and T. K. Sundaresan, *Resource Allocation Model for Public Health Planning: A Case Study of Tuberculosis Control*, World Health Organization, Geneva, 1973.
2. See Jaime Rodriguez and Jesus Rico, eds., *Componentes Evaluativos de la Atencion Primaria*, PRIMOPS document, Cali, Colombia, 1977, for a discussion of the relative time required by alternative outpatient services. This information was supplemented by unpublished reports for the Antonio Narino and Luis H. Garces health centers.

Chapter 7

Stimulation with the Model

INTRODUCTION

Before considering the results of the optimization analysis it is useful to review a series of simulation experiments designed to illuminate characteristics of the model and to underline some important considerations in the choice of health activities to reduce child mortality. All of the simulations reported here are based on the morbidity and usage coefficients and fatality rates derived from the full set of responses obtained in the survey of professional opinion. The simulations produce the marginal and joint disease rates and mortality rates that are the consequence of given sets of activity levels. The first section of the chapter gives the results of a simulation using the baseline activity levels. For comparison, and to calculate the operational range of the effects of the activities, the second section gives the results of simulations using, alternatively, a zero-level activity set and a maximum-level activity set. A demonstration of the importance of promoting usage is given in the third section. The effects of the disease interaction terms are considered in the fourth section. Demonstration of the interrelationship between preventive activities and the cost of curative care is given in the fifth section. The final section of the chapter demonstrates some difficulties that may arise in the use of single simulations to form piecewise estimates of the cost effectiveness of separate activities and underlines the importance of using an optimization or programming procedure to find the best choice of activities levels.

Table 7–1. Baseline Simulation Results.

	0–1 Month Age Group	*1–12 Month Age Group*	*12–60 Month Age Group*
I. Marginal morbidity rates			
Low birth weight	.100		
Infection	.150		
Birth trauma	.040		
Tetanus	.005		
Malnutrition		.100	.150
Diarrhea		.170	.110
Respiratory		.060	.020
Immunizable		.005	.004
II. Joint morbidity rates			
Tetanus, all states	.005		
Low birth weight only	.063		
Birth trauma only	.031		
Infection only	.109		
Low birth weight & birth trauma	.003		
Birth trauma & infection	.032		
Low birth weight & infection	.005		
Low birth weight & birth trauma & infection	.001		
Malnutrition only		.0003	.0517
Diarrhea only		.0786	.0251
Respiratory only		.0384	.0064
Immunizable only		.0039	.0009
Malnutrition & immunizable		.0050	.0027
Malnutrition & diarrhea		.0804	.0824
Malnutrition & respiratory		.0112	.0108
Other combinations		.0107	.0026
III. Fatality rates			
Tetanus, all states	.881		
Low birth rate only	.165		
Birth trauma only	.220		
Infection only	.028		
Low birth weight & birth trauma	.333		
Low birth weight & infection	.274		
Birth trauma & infection	.227		
Low birth weight & birth trauma & infection	.388		
Malnutrition only		.0055	.0027
Diarrhea only		.0060	.0017
Respiratory only		.0124	.0026
Immunizable only		.0042	.0267
Malnutrition & immunizable		.1443	.0487
Malnutrition & diarrhea		.0189	.0063
Malnutrition & respiratory		.0238	.0055
Other combinations		.0466	.0217

Table 7–1. *(Continued)*

	0–1 Month Age Group	*1–12 Month Age Group*	*12–60 Month Age Group*
IV. Usage rates			
Prenatal care, all women	.10		
Prenatal care, pregnant women	.12		
Curative care, neonatal	.20		
Breast feeding	.30	.30	
Early prenatal care	.12		
Preventive care, infant		.10	
Curative care, infant		.20	
Preventive care, toddler			.10
Curative care, toddler			.20
V. Age group mortality rate[a]	.045	.060	.062
Number of survivors[b]			10596

[a] The age group mortality rate per population and period covered by the age group.
[b] The maximum potential number of survivors, assuming that the mortality rate in each age group is zero, is 12,462.

SIMULATION USING THE BASELINE ACTIVITY SET

The baseline activity set produces the patterns of morbidity summarized in Table 7–1. The rates generated are, of course, identical with the baseline morbidity rates used to calculate the coefficients. The result of the low level of baseline activities is a high level of mortality; the neonatal, infant, and early childhood mortality rates[a] are 45, 60, and 62, respectively, and the number of survivors is only 10,596 out of a maximum total of 12,462.

Given the respondents' opinions of the importance of disease interaction, the baseline marginal disease rates generate the joint morbidity rates listed in section II of Table 7–1. A perusal of the joint disease rates reveals that malnutrition (of grades II and III) is very likely to occur in combination with another disease in the last two age groups. This is especially important for the infant age group where it is found that essentially all severe malnutrition is found in combination with other diseases, particularly diarrhea. Because the baseline proportion of population receiving curative care is low, the baseline fatality rates are high, especially for disease categories where malnutrition is involved. The result is that a high proportion of mortality occurs where malnutrition is present. It is of

[a] Note that as used in this study "infant mortality rate" refers to the number of deaths of children 1–12 months old per 1000 children in the 1–12 month age group.

interest to compare these simulation results with actual data to see if the pattern of mortality generated by the model is reflective of reality.

The comparison is made by looking at the pattern of mortality revealed by the Puffer and Serrano study[1] for the Cali, Recife, and suburban San Juan samples. Difficulties are introduced by the fact that the PAHO study is based on random samples covering a citywide population base that, especially for Cali, may not be precisely reflective of the morbidity and mortality conditions in a low-income *barrio*. The Recife and San Juan samples were chosen as more representative of the conditions being modeled than the other samples used in the PAHO study. An additional problem of comparison is introduced by the difficulty of reclassifying the diseases cited as associated or underlying causes of mortality in the PAHO study into the categories used by the child mortality model. The disease categories used in the model are, however, defined broadly and, except for the birth trauma and neonatal infection categories, the classification problem may not be severe.

Table 7–2. Comparison of Cause of Mortality, from Baseline Simulation and Puffer and Serrano Study.

Underlying or Associated Cause	*Percent of Total Mortality*		
	Simulation		*Puffer and Serrano*[a]
0–28 days	No tetanus	With tetanus	
low birth weight	53	48	58–65
infection	35	32	21–27
birth trauma	25	22	21–22[b]
tetanus	—	10	—
1–12 months			
malnutrition		52	48–61
diarrhea		49	56–75
respiratory		24	15–31
immunizable		22	5–9
12–60 months			
malnutrition		69	42–57
diarrhea		51	60–70
respiratory		11	9–15
immunizable		14	20–30

[a] Rates given are based on Cali, Recife, and San Juan samples from Ruth Puffer and Carlos Serrano, eds., *Patterns of Mortality in Childhood*, Pan American Health Organization, Scientific Publication, No. 262, Washington, D.C., 1973. Some error in deriving comparable figures from the PAHO study may have been introduced by the necessity of arbitrarily classifying the diseases enumerated by Puffer and Serrano into the categories used by the child mortality model. This problem is especially important for the neonatal infection and birth trauma categories.

[b] "Certain perinatal causes of death" (not including low birth weight, hemolytic disease, or congenital abnormalities).

The comparison, shown in Table 7–2, reveals that the pattern of mortality from the model corresponds to a considerable extent with the pattern found by the PAHO study. The PAHO study confirms the importance of malnutrition as an associated cause of mortality and an ordering of the causes of mortality in each group is the same in both cases with the exception of diarrhea in the last two age groups. The major discrepancy between the two distributions is that diarrhea, although involved in 50 percent of mortality in the model, differs by 10 to 25 percent from the Puffer and Serrano study.

It would, of course, be possible to "tune" the model by altering the baseline morbidity and fatality rates and the interaction coefficients to reproduce the exact pattern revealed by the PAHO study. However, given the difficulties in classifying mortality by cause and the possible lack of comparability between the communities in the PAHO study and the hypothetical low-income community being modeled, it is not clear that such adjustment would be an improvement and it was decided to leave the model parameters unaltered. Instead, the extent of correspondence between the two patterns of mortality is interpreted as a confirmation of the operational realism of the simulation model.

SIMULATIONS USING THE MINIMUM AND MAXIMUM ACTIVITY SETS

When all activities are set at a zero level, the morbidity and mortality rates implied by the model are as given in Table 7–3. These rates are the maximum that results, given the baseline socioeconomic characteristics of the population, from a total lack of health activity. Under these least favorable conditions, the model implies a neonatal mortality rate of 51 per 1000 births, a mortality rate for the infant age group of 70 per 1000, and a mortality rate of 78 per 1000 in early childhood. The number of survivors to an age of sixty months is only 10,129 out of a potential number of survivors of 12,462. These rates provide a useful reference with which to gauge the simulated improvement to be derived from selected nonzero sets of activities.

Looking at the opposite extreme, Table 7–4 gives the resulting rates of morbidity and mortality if all thirty-two activities are set at the maximum possible levels. At the maximum levels, given by the demographic and epidemiological constraints, there is total coverage of the relevant target population groups for each activity and the mortality rates generated are a minimum for the model (again holding the socioeconomic variables constant). Under these most favorable conditions, the number of survivors is 11,963 and the neonatal, infant, and early childhood rates are 12, 13, and 15

Table 7–3. Simulation Using Minimum Activity Set (100% usage assumed).

	0–1 Month Age Group	1–12 Month Age Group	12–60 Month Age Group
I. Marginal morbidity rates			
Low birth weight	.109		
Infection	.205		
Birth trauma	.044		
Tetanus	.006		
Malnutrition		.137	.173
Diarrhea		.236	.148
Respiratory		.070	.022
Immunizable		.005	.004
II. Joint morbidity rates			
Tetanus, all states	.006		
Low birth weight only	.063		
Birth trauma only	.032		
Infection only	.154		
Low birth weight & birth trauma	.003		
Low birth weight & infection	.041		
Birth trauma & infection	.007		
Low birth weight & birth trauma & infection	.002		
Malnutrition only		.0026	.0500
Diarrhea only		.1010	.0398
Respiratory only		.0404	.0065
Immunizable only		.0039	.0009
Malnutrition & immunizable		.0007	.0031
Malnutrition & diarrhea		.1082	.1047
Malnutrition & respiratory		.0134	.0115
Other combinations		.0164	.0035
III. Fatality rates			
Tetanus, all states	.910		
Low birth rate only	.178		
Birth trauma only	.230		
Infection only	.031		
Low birth weight & birth trauma	.350		
Low birth weight & infection	.293		
Birth trauma & infection	.293		
Low birth weight & birth trauma & infection	.408		
Malnutrition only		.0060	.0030
Diarrhea only		.0070	.0020
Respiratory only		.0140	.0030
Immunizable only		.0790	.0290
Malnutrition & immunizable		.1540	.0530
Malnutrition & diarrhea		.0210	.0070
Malnutrition & respiratory		.0260	.0060
Other combinations		.0500	.0240
IV. Age group mortality rate	.051	.070	.078
Number of survivors			10129

Table 7–4. Simulation Using Maximum Activity Set (100% usage assumed).

	0–1 Month Age Group	*1–12 Month Age Group*	*12–60 Month Age Group*
I. Marginal morbidity rates			
Low birth weight	.029		
Infection	.053		
Birth trauma	.020		
Tetanus	.000		
Malnutrition		.010	.012
Diarrhea		.019	.022
Respiratory		.032	.008
Immunizable		.001	.0004
II. Joint morbidity rates			
Tetanus, all states	.000		
Low birth weight only	.021		
Birth trauma only	.019		
Infection only	.044		
Low birth weight & birth trauma	.000		
Low birth weight & infection	.007		
Birth trauma & infection	.001		
Low birth weight & birth trauma & infection	.000		
Malnutrition only		.0000	.0000
Diarrhea only		.0093	.0108
Respiratory only		.0285	.0062
Immunizable only		.0006	.0001
Malnutrition & immunizable		.0000	.0002
Malnutrition & diarrhea		.0086	.0115
Malnutrition & respiratory		.0031	.0014
Other combinations		.0006	.0003
III. Fatality rates			
Tetanus, all states	.448		
Low birth rate only	.080		
Birth trauma only	.124		
Infection only	.010		
Low birth weight & birth trauma	.185		
Low birth weight & infection	.133		
Birth trauma & infection	.142		
Low birth weight & birth trauma & infection	.236		
Malnutrition only		.0024	.0008
Diarrhea only		.0014	.0003
Respiratory only		.0035	.0005
Immunizable only		.0297	.0107
Malnutrition & immunizable		.0600	.0197
Malnutrition & diarrhea		.0075	.0022
Malnutrition & respiratory		.0099	.0021
Other combinations		.0177	.0065
IV. Age group mortality rate	.012	.013	.015
Number of survivors			11963

Table 7–5. Range of Morbidity and Mortality Between Minimum and Maximum Activity Levels.

	0–1 Month Age Group	*1–12 Month Age Group*	*12–60 Month Age Group*
I. Marginal morbidity rates			
Low birth weight	.008		
Infection	.152		
Birth trauma	.024		
Tetanus	.006		
Malnutrition		.127	.161
Diarrhea		.207	.126
Respiratory		.038	.014
Immunizable		.004	.0036
II. Age group mortality rates	.039	.057	.063
III. Number of survivors			1834

per 1000. These rates provide the upper limit on the number of survivors, obtainable only with a resource expenditure several times the quantity of resources presently available to the community.

Comparing the two extremes, it is seen that the difference in the number of survivors is 1834, which is a measure of the range or latitude over which changes in the control variables (the thirty-two activities) can influence the extent of mortality. An examination of Table 7–5 reveals that between the two extremes neonatal mortality falls by 39 per 1000 births, infant mortality by 57 per 1000, and mortality in early childhood falls by 60 per 1000. In percentage terms, neonatal mortality falls by 74 percent and infant and early childhood mortality by 81 percent. The greatest part of this improvement results from reductions in the morbidity rates for low birth weight, malnutrition, and diarrhea, a fact that anticipates some of the results to be demonstrated in the following chapter on optimum resource allocation.

THE IMPORTANCE OF PROMOTIONAL ACTIVITIES

The maximum possible number of survivors is calculated under the assumption that all activities made available are used if needed by the respective target populations. In actuality, although a need for the activities may exist, available activities may go unused because mothers are unaware of health needs or are insufficiently motivated to use available services. Table 7–6 presents a demonstration of the importance of motivating the use of health services. The table gives the impact of prenatal

Table 7–6. An Illustration of the Importance of Promotional Activities.

	No Promotora or Mass Media		*With Promotora and Mass Media*	
	Prenatal Care Activities Set at Maximum[a]	*Nutritional Activities Set at Maximum*[b]	*Prenatal Care Activities Set at Maximum*[a]	*Nutritional Activities Set at Maximum*[b]
I. Marginal morbidity rates				
0–1 age group				
Low birth weight	.099	.105	.040	.070
Infection	.180	.187	.093	.128
Birth trauma	.043	.043	.037	.043
Tetanus	.005	.006	.000	.005
1–12 age group				
Malnutrition	.1155	.1121	.0569	.0560
Diarrhea	.2076	.2068	.1293	.1291
Respiratory	.0638	.0635	.0512	.0511
Immunizable	.0050	.0050	.0045	.0045
12–60 age group				
Malnutrition	.1693	.1622	.0902	.0505
Diarrhea	.1474	.1456	.1036	.0937
Respiratory	.0218	.0212	.0160	.0132
Immunizable	.0044	.0043	.0036	.0032
II. Usage rates				
Prenatal care, preg. women	.12	.12	.95	.95
Early prenatal care	.12	.12	.95	.95
Preventive care, 1–12	.10	.10	.93	.93
Preventive care, 12–60	.10	.10	.96	.96
Breast feeding	.30	.30	.80	.80
III. Age group mortality rates				
0–1	.047	.050	.027	.039
1–12	.064	.063	.045	.045
12–60	.077	.076	.053	.043
IV. Number of survivors	10247	10247	10956	10935

[a] Activities providing prenatal care for pregnant women, $X(3)$, $X(7)$ through $X(11)$, are set at maximum levels. Other activities are set at zero except for promotora and mass media, which are set at maximum or zero as indicated by the column heading.

[b] Nutritional programs for pregnant women, $X(11)$, children 1–12 months, $X(25)$ and children 12–60 months, $X(30)$, are set at maximum. All other activities are set at zero except for promotora and mass media, which are set at maximum or minimum levels as indicated by the column heading.

Table 7–7. Impact of Selected Activities with All Other Activities at Zero Level (100% usage assumed).

	0–1 Month Age Group	*1–12 Month Age Group*	*12–60 Month Age Group*
I. Nutritional activities[a]			
A. Marginal morbidity rates			
Low birth weight	.082		
Infection	.199		
Birth trauma	.044		
Tetanus	.006		
Malnutrition		.099	.090
Diarrhea		.217	.127
Respiratory		.066	.015
Immunizable		.005	.004
B. Mortality rates	.045	.064	.057
C. Number of survivors			10495
II. Piped water in all homes[b]			
A. Marginal morbidity rates			
Low birth weight	.103		
Infection	.165		
Birth trauma	.044		
Tetanus	.006		
Malnutrition		.116	.152
Diarrhea		.170	.102
Respiratory		.068	.021
Immunizable		.005	.004
B. Mortality rates	.048	.060	.067
C. Number of survivors			10393
III. Early prenatal care[c]			
A. Marginal morbidity rates			
Low birth weight	.045		
Infection	.147		
Birth trauma	.037		
Tetanus	.000		
Malnutrition		.130	.172
Diarrhea		.225	.148
Respiratory		.069	.022
Immunizable		.005	.004
B. Mortality rates	.029	.069	.078
C. Number of survivors			10377

Table 7–7. *(Continued)*

	0–1 Month Age Group	*1–12 Month Age Group*	*12–60 Month Age Group*
IV. Promotora and mass media[d]			
A. Marginal morbidity rates			
Low birth weight	.092		
Infection	.133		
Birth trauma	.044		
Tetanus	.055		
Malnutrition		.063	.091
Diarrhea		.131	.104
Respiratory		.052	.016
Immunizable		.005	.004
B. Mortality rates	.044	.046	.054
C. Number of survivors			10752

[a] *X*(11), *X*(25), and *X*(30) at maximum level.
[b] *X*(18) at maximum level.
[c] *X*(3), *X*(7), *X*(8), *X*(9), *X*(10), and *X*(11) at maximum level.
[d] *X*(1) and *X*(22) at maximum level.

care activities and nutritional programs; a measure of the impact of the programs can be obtained by comparing the mortality rates and number of survivors with the maximum rates and minimum number of survivors calculated using the zero activity set. Without a promotora or mass media program only 10 percent of available intervention capacity is used and the increase in the number of survivors (NOS) is only 118. This is less than half the increase in the number of survivors that would be expected to accompany full use of the selected nutritional or prenatal care programs (see Table 7–7).

With promotora and mass media programs, the use of the health activities increases to approximately 95 percent and the benefit from the nutritional and prenatal care programs is much greater. In addition, the promotora and mass media activities carry their own direct benefits (summarized in part IV of Table 7–7) that have substantial impacts, primarily through nutritional education and increased breast feeding, on the morbidity rates for malnutrition and diarrhea. The combined result of the promotional and either prenatal care or nutritional programs is an increase in the number of survivors of approximately 800.

The use of well-baby clinics, health system deliveries, immunizations, and outpatient and inpatient care is also affected by the level of promotora and mass media activities. Because the promotion activities are relatively low in cost, yet have the important effect of regulating the usage of most of the activities considered in the model, it can be expected that they will be assigned a prominent role by the optimization program.

DISEASE INTERDEPENDENCE

Many of the activities not only affect morbidity through a direct attack on the primary conditions or health environment underlying the development of disease but also affect morbidity indirectly through a reduction of associated diseases. Although the direct effects are the largest part of the total impact of the activities, the indirect effects are considerable. Inclusion of the disease interaction terms allows the model to capture the indirect effects of activities. It will be recalled from Figure 3–1 and the associated discussion that the indirect effects included in the model are between diseases in each age group, especially between diarrhea and malnutrition, as well as across age groups for low birth weight and malnutrition.

By considering the impact of specific sets of activities that have direct effects only on single diseases, we can examine changes in associated diseses to obtain some indication of the importance of the disease interaction terms. To do this we calculate the change in selected disease rates and number of survivors with and without the set of activities under consideration, all other activities being kept at zero level. The change in the morbidity rates with an introduction of selected interventions is calculated using two alternative simulation models; the first uses the full set of estimated coefficients and the second uses the same coefficients with the exclusion of the interaction terms.

An example of the effect of interactions among diseases within age groups is given by considering the impact of 100 percent participation of pregnant women, infants, and children between twelve and sixty months in the nutrition programs. As policy variables, these activities enter directly only in the low-birth-weight and malnutrition functions. With all interaction coefficients omitted and all other activities except the nutritional programs kept at a zero level, the impact of the nutritional activities is to increase the number of survivors by 220. The low-birth-weight rate is reduced by 0.028 and the malnutrition rates are reduced by 0.032 and 0.069; all other morbidity rates remain unchanged. With interaction coefficients included, the change in the number of survivors is 367 and the morbidity rate for diarrhea is reduced by 0.009 in the infant age group and by 0.021 in the early childhood age group. There are further small reductions in low birth weight and malnutrition due to the feedback effects of the disease interaction.

Table 7–8. Change in Morbidity Rates and Number of Survivors with Selected Activities and with and without Disease Interaction.

	With Interaction Terms			*Without Interaction Terms*		
Selected Diseases	*Nutritional Programs*	*Piped Water*	*Prenatal Care*	*Nutritional Programs*	*Piped Water*	*Prenatal Care*
0–28 days						
Low birth weight	.028	.008	.075	.028	.008	.065
Infection	.006	.040	.058	—	.039	.045
1–12 months						
Malnutrition	.038	.021	.007	.032	—	—
Diarrhea	.009	.056	.001	—	.052	—
12–60 months						
Malnutrition	.083	.021	.001	.069	—	—
Diarrhea	.021	.046	—	—	.041	—
Number of survivors	367	265	249	220	145	230

The indirect effects of water and sanitation are also substantial. With all other activities kept at a zero level, the direct impact of supplying piped water to 100 percent of the households is to reduce diarrhea in the last two age groups by 0.052 and 0.041 and to increase the number of survivors by 145. When disease interaction is included, the simulated impact is to increase the number of survivors by 265. The indirect effects on the rate of malnutrition are substantial. The rate for malnutrition in the infant and early childhood period is reduced by 0.021 by the indirect impact of the water program.

In contrast to the large indirect effects simulated for the nutritional and water activities, the indirect effects of prenatal care activities are much less substantial. In this case the effects are carried across age groups by the link between low birth weight and malnutrition. Because the linking coefficient is estimated to be small, the reduction in malnutrition in the infant age group is only 0.007 and the reduction in the early childhood period is negligible. The indirect effects across age groups are, therefore, not as important an aspect of the model as the indirect effects among diseases within age groups. The indirect effects of both water and nutritional activities are significant, however, and the examples given above illustrate that interdependence among diseases can be an important component in an evaluation of the impact of specific activities.

THE COST OF CURATIVE CARE UNDER ALTERNATIVE MORBIDITY CONDITIONS

Simulations with the model demonstrate that the cost of providing treatment for all ill children varies considerably with the level of preventive activities. As the level of preventive activities increases, morbidity rates fall reducing the cost of treating a given percentage of all morbidity. When preventive activities are at a minimum and morbidity rates are at a maximum, as shown in Table 7–4, the cost of covering 100 percent of the population with inpatient care is 10,967,289 pesos (which is well beyond the resources available to the community). With preventive activities at a level sufficient to cover one-half of the relevant population groups, the level of morbidity falls and the cost of 100 percent coverage by inpatient care falls to 4,620,413 pesos, and with full coverage by preventive care, the level of morbidity (see Table 7–3) falls sufficiently that 100-percent coverage by inpatient care costs only 1,656,718 pesos—approximately 15 percent of the cost when there is a total lack of preventive care. A similar outcome, shown in Table 7–9, is obtained for outpatient care.

As a result of the interaction between morbidity and the cost of curative care, a level of coverage with curative care that is infeasible in the absence of preventive activities becomes a possibility in combination with preventive care. Given its high cost, it is likely that inpatient care will not be a cost-effective activity unless the resources of the community are sufficiently great to also allow a high level of preventive care. However, the relatively lower cost of outpatient care, together with the reduction in the morbidity base, opens the possibility that given a judicious choice of

Table 7–9. Cost of Providing Curative Treatment under Alternative Morbidity Conditions.

	Total Morbidity Requiring Treatment (# of cases/28 days)			*Cost of Treating All Cases*[b] *(Colombian pesos)*	
Level of Preventive Activities[a]	*0–1 Months*	*1–12 Months*	*12–60 Months*	*Inpatient Care*	*Outpatient Care*
Zero level	73	800	2,586	10,967,289	463,357
Half level	41	390	1,014	4,620,413	193,111
Full level	22	138	356	1,656,718	68,586

[a] The level of all preventive activities $X(1) \ldots X(13)$, $X(18) \ldots X(26)$, $X(29)$, and $X(30)$ are set to their respective maximum epidemiological and demographic levels.

[b] For reference, recall from Chapter 6 that the total peso budget available to the community for child health care is 2,591,344.

preventive activities, outpatient care *may* be a cost-effective activity even at relatively modest levels of resources. To determine whether this is true or not must await the optimization results in Chapter 8.

MARGINAL COST EFFECTIVENESS AND ACTIVITY LEVELS

Marginal cost effectiveness (MCE) of a given activity can be defined as the change in the number of survivors with a change in the expenditure on the activity. Marginal cost effectiveness can be calculated by dividing the impact on the number of survivors accompanying a given change in activity level by the cost of the increase in the activity. In the present model, the costs per unit of activity are constant, so that whether marginal cost effectiveness is decreasing, constant, or increasing depends on the characteristics of the morbidity functions that determine the marginal impact of the activities. Given the shape of the logit function used in the simulation, it is apparent that any of the three alternatives are possible.[b] For instance, *at a zero level* for all other activities, the MCE of only a nutrition or only a prenatal care program is slightly decreasing; the MCE of immunizations or curative care programs is constant; the MCE of water, sanitation, or promotora programs is very slightly increasing.

As the level of expenditure on all other activities increases, the MCE of any given activity declines markedly. Figure 7–1 illustrates this effect for water programs. At low levels for all other activities, the marginal cost effectiveness of increases in a water activity is given by $MCE^{I}_{H_2O}$. As the level of other programs (notably those affecting neonatal infection and diarrhea) increases, the relationship between MCE and scale of activity of water programs declines as given by the successive MCE_{H_2O} curves.

Thus, a general feature of the model, that is probably an apt reflection of reality, is the marked decline in the marginal cost effectiveness that accompanies an increase in expenditure on a given activity as the level of expenditure on all other activities increases. Simulations with the model demonstrate that the change in the number of survivors with an increase in all activities from a level of zero to half of the demographic maximum is 1639, whereas the change in the number of survivors as activities increase from half level to full level is only 195. As a consequence, the average cost of increasing the number of survivors by one increases from 3,722 pesos to

[b] The characteristics of the logit function for a given disease depend on the baseline data, the importance of the socioeconomic variables (SES variables are kept constant throughout this analysis but they nevertheless play a role in determining the constant term in the logit function), and the upper and lower bounds on the function.

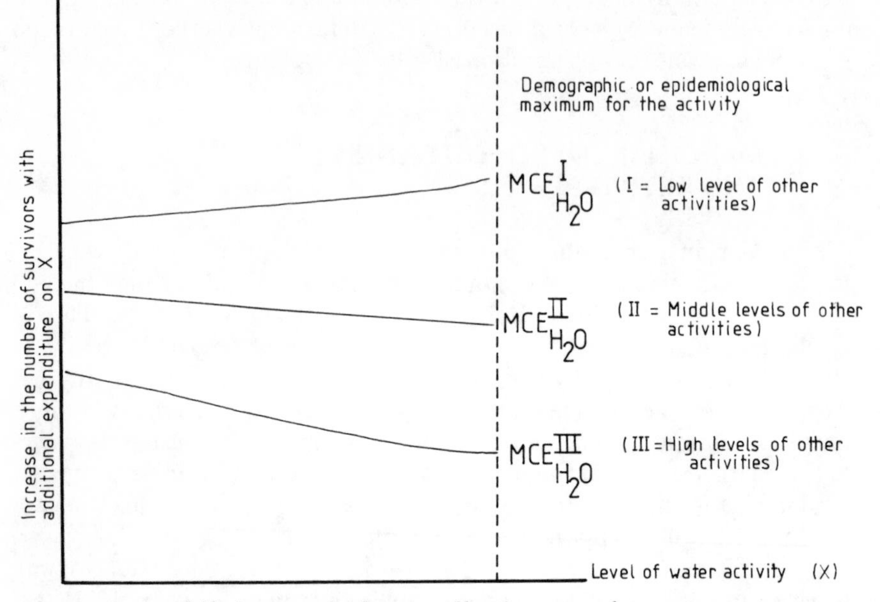

Figure 7–1. Shift in marginal cost effectiveness of a water program as the level of other activities increases.

31,282 pesos between the two cases. This result is reported only to emphasize the extent of diminishing returns to additional expenditure in the model. In actuality, of course, a simple rule such as setting all activities at an equal fraction of full level would lead to a costly, suboptimal use of resources. For instance, commencing at an initial level of zero, there are many activities that will increase the number of survivors by one for less than 3,722 pesos (or for less than 31,282 pesos when all other activities are at half of full level).

Because of the continuing shift in the MCE of given activities as the levels of other activities change, it is possible that activities that are relatively cost effective at one resource level will be relatively cost ineffective at another level. For example, at a zero level for all other activities, the marginal cost effectiveness of immunizations is as indicated by MCE^{I}_{IMM} in Figure 7–2. As expenditure increases on activities other than immunizations, the morbidity rate for immunizable disease falls and the marginal cost effectiveness of preventing mortality by inoculation decreases, say, to MCE^{II}_{IMM} as the risk of contracting an immunizable disease is reduced. A tempting conclusion might be, then, that immunizations are,

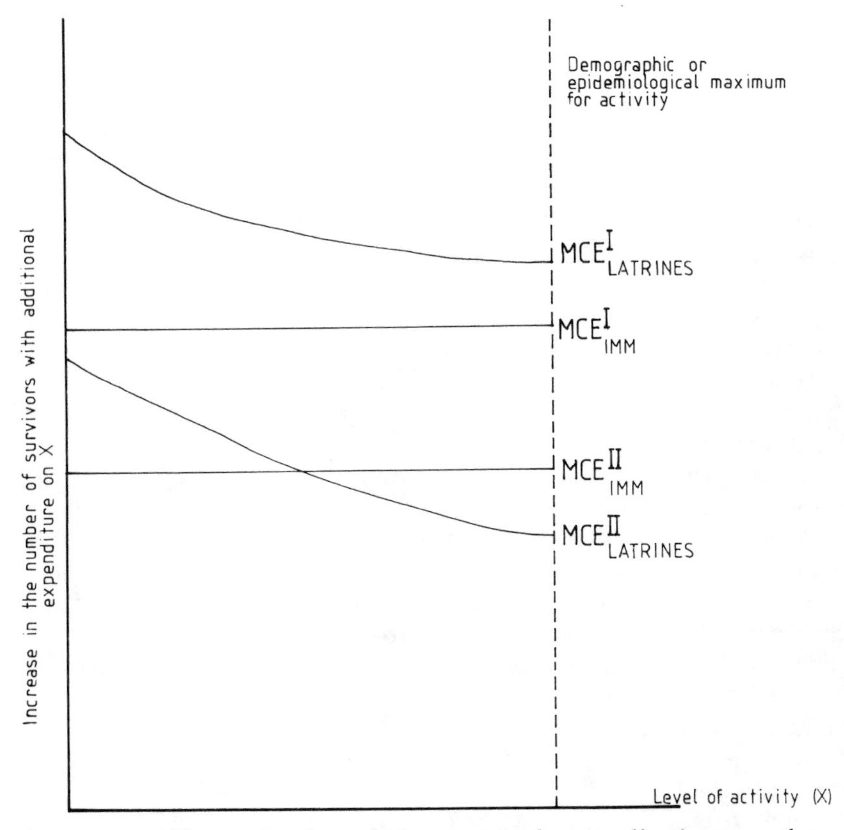

Figure 7–2. Change in the relative marginal cost effectiveness of two activities as the general level of all activities increases (from I to II).

relative to other activities, cost effective at low resource levels and less so at high resource levels, but this is not confirmed by the model. Continuing with Figure 7–2, we see that the marginal impact of other activities declines even faster at high resource levels and that, for instance, the marginal cost effectiveness of latrines is greater than that of immunizations at low resource levels but less at high resource levels. Clearly, a simple piecewise comparison of the relative cost effectiveness of alternative interventions that does not consider the simultaneous level of other interventions can be misleading. The optimization procedure applied in Chapter 8 allows a consideration of the simultaneous impact of interventions and provides a selection of the most cost effective *set* of interventions for given resource levels.

SUMMARY

This chapter uses simulations based on alternative activity sets to explore the characteristics of the model. A simulation with the model using baseline activity levels for the hypothetical community produces a distribution of mortality by cause of death that is in accord with the pattern of mortality reported for actual communities in the PAHO study by Puffer and Serrano.[2] Simulations using minimum (zero level) and maximum (total coverage of relevant demographic groups) activity levels show that the possible range between the worst and best possible activity sets is 1834 survivors. In terms of infant mortality the range is from 120/1000 births to 25/1000 births. The simulations show that the greatest part of the reduction in mortality comes from reducing the morbidity rates for diarrhea and malnutrition.

Another set of simulations demonstrates that the interactions between diseases can be important, especially the interaction between malnutrition and diarrhea. Promotion is shown to play a key role in the model, acting as a valve that regulates the use of available activities. In addition the direct effects of the promotora and the impact of increased breast feeding on diarrhea and malnutrition are substantial. These direct effects are magnified by the indirect effect of disease interaction. The general decrease in morbidity that accompanies increased preventive care significantly reduces the level of curative care needed to cover the population adequately. At low levels of preventive care, the level of curative care required to treat all morbidity is financially infeasible; with higher levels of preventive care, curative care becomes a practical possibility.

A general feature of the model is the diminished marginal cost effectiveness of any given activity as the level of other activities increases. The cross impact between the effectiveness of one activity and the level of another makes it particularly difficult to examine the cost effectiveness of separate activities out of the context of other associated health activities. This provides a strong reason for the use of an optimization model that considers the cost effectiveness of a joint set of activities.

NOTES

1. Ruth Puffer and Carlos Serrano, eds., *Patterns of Mortality in Childhood*, Pan American Health Organization, Scientific Publication No. 262, Washington, D.C., 1973.
2. *Ibid.*

Chapter 8

Optimization with the Model

INTRODUCTION

The allocation of resources that will maximize the proportion of children surviving through the first sixty months of life cannot easily be determined by inspection of either the costs or impacts of the alternative health activities. Disease interactions, the distinction between usage and availability, variations in the relative impact of interventions with variations in resource levels, and activities that have direct effects on more than one disease and in more than one age group all add complexities that are likely to exist in most developing communities. These complications make it unlikely that a direct solution to the optimization problem could be obtained by simple experiments with single runs of the simulation model. Instead, a systematic procedure is needed to sort through the possibilities and find the optimum solution.

This chapter reports the results of using a nonlinear computer optimization program to provide such a systematic sorting of the possible solutions to obtain a selection of optimum levels for the set of activities. In order to provide the background necessary for an assessment of the optimal solutions, the first section of the chapter contains a short discussion of the optimization procedure. This section points out some limitations of the optimization technique that qualify the solutions obtained. The second section examines the optimal solution for a reference run using the level of resource constraints that is most likely to apply to the baseline hypothetical community being modeled. The third section examines changes in the optimum activity mix with changes in the general level of resource constraints. Put somewhat differently, this section attempts to discern changes in the relative importance of health activities as all resources become uniformly more abundant. The final section looks at the value of increasing individual resources that were exhausted in the optimal solutions discussed in the previous sections.

THE OPTIMIZATION PROCEDURE

As a general rule, it is easier to find an optimum for a linear than for a nonlinear problem. The problem at hand is, however, nonlinear and, although the nonlinearity adds considerably to the realism and interest of the model, it also adds some difficulties in obtaining and interpreting optimal solutions. The computer program used is EXPLORE and was written by Byron S. Gottfried.[1] The program is intended to solve nonlinear optimization problems where the independent variables (in our case, the alternative health activities) vary continuously within a set of lower and upper bounds (in our case, the zero activity levels and demographic constraints provide the bounds). Because unconstrained optimal problems are easier to solve than constrained problems, EXPLORE operates by assigning penalty values to the violation of constraints—the magnitude of the penalty being a power of the extent of the violation. The penalties are added to the objective (number of survivors) and a gradient search procedure is used to find the optimum of the modified and unconstrained objective function. In practice, the penalties for violation of the constraints are large enough that optimization tends to drive the penalties to zero, satisfying the constraints. An iterative search procedure is used that continues as long as the gradients for alternative independent variables (activity levels) are positive and as long as the objective continues to be improved by a proportional change greater than a prespecified value, ε.

Continuous problems with a single mode or optimum such as that of finding the maximum of Y with respect to X in Figure 8–1,[a] are handled efficiently by the EXPLORE algorithms. Given a point at which to start the search, such as X_0, the program discovers that improvements in the

[a] Figures 8–1 through 8–3 are intended to give heuristic descriptions using only a single independent variable, of some of the difficulties to be met in finding an optimal solution to a nonlinear problem. The actual problem to be considered is, of course, multidimensional and cannot be depicted in a diagram.

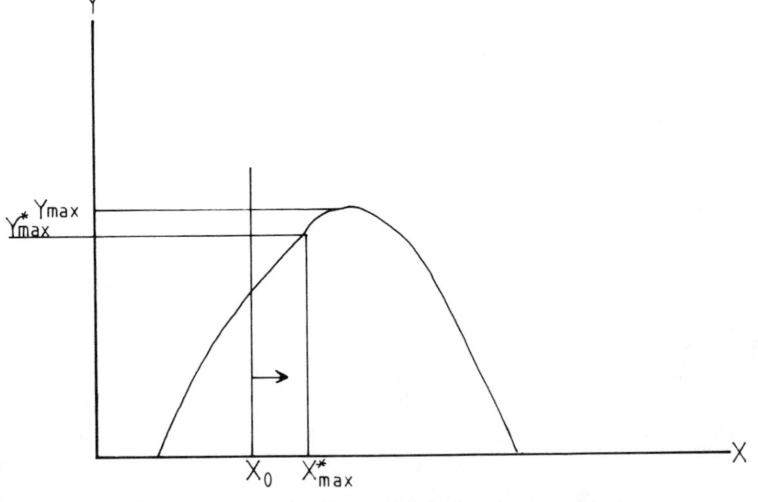

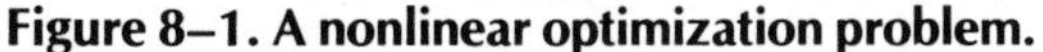
Figure 8–1. A nonlinear optimization problem.

objective, Y, can be obtained by moving in the direction of the arrow towards X^*_{max}. A possible solution is found at Y^*_{max}, which differs (but only slightly) from Y_{max}.

But the child mortality model is multimodal and may contain local optimal solutions as well as a global optimum. This problem is depicted in two dimensions in Figure 8–2. Now, when the computer program starts at

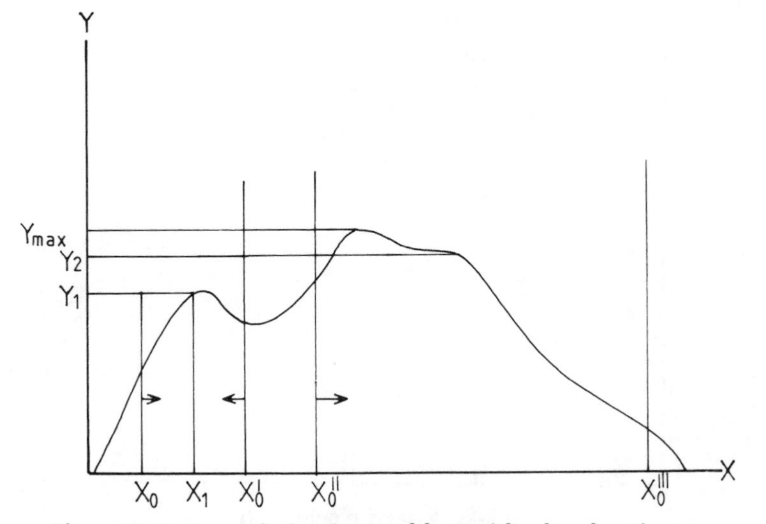

Figure 8–2. An optimization problem with a local optimum.

X_0 and moves in the direction of a positive gradient, the program finds a possible solution at Y_1 with activity level X_1 although the global optimum is at Y_{max}. Another problem that may exist is that the search may be stopped when a plateau is reached that gives improvements in the objective that are smaller than epsilon as at Y_2 in Figure 8–2. These problems are attacked by using a "grid" of alternative starting points such as X_0, X_0', X_0'', and X_0'''. In this example X_0'' leads to the discovery of Y_{max}.

In practice the use of a grid search when the number of activities is large is impractical and only a coarse grid was used on the child mortality problem. A coarse grid raises the possibility that a needle peak, such as at *A* in Figure 8–3, might be missed. This is not an important problem with the model at hand, however, since the narrower the band of *X* values encompassing the peak the more difficult and subject to error would be the implementation of the precise policies needed to achieve the optimum. It is more likely, given the broad ranges over which the morbidity functions are continuous and monotonic,[b] that the child survival optimization problem does not contain "needle peak" solutions. In any case, our interest is in more stable, broad based solutions that are less sensitive to policy error such as at *B*, rather than *A*, in Figure 8–3.

[b] Monotonic denotes that the sign of the change in the dependent variable with a change in an independent variable remains the same throughout the range of the function. The individual functions making up the separate components of the model are all monotonic. A possibility of discontinuities and nonmonotonic behavior is introduced by the selection of the minimum of usage or availability in determining the intervention variables used as arguments in the morbidity and fatality functions.

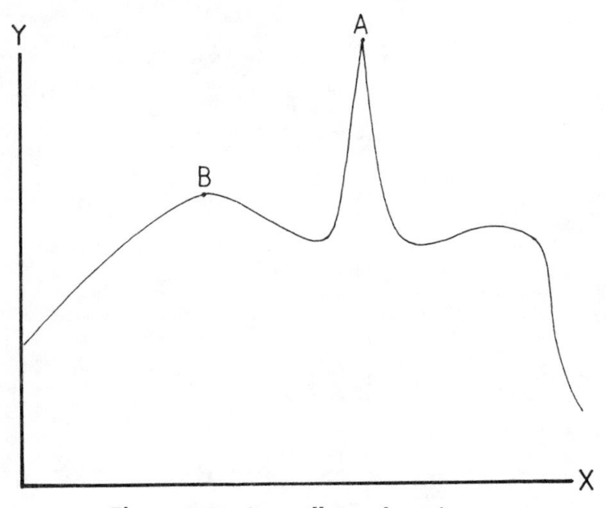

Figure 8–3. A needle peak optimum.

The operational qualifications to the possible optimum discovered by the computer program are, then: (1) the program may stop on a plateau after experiment shows that improvement greater than ε is not possible; and (2) local optima may exist that preclude the discovery of the global solution. As a matter of mathematical rigor, the solution is called a "possible" optimum because it cannot rigorously be established that the program has indeed turned up the very best allocation of resources. But as a practical matter the allocation produced by the program is probably capable of only small improvement.

OPTIMUM ALLOCATION OF RESOURCES IN THE MODELED COMMUNITY

As a reference, we examine the optimum allocation of resources and activity levels when all resource constraints are set at 0.75 of the full level of resources estimated in Chapter 6 to be available to the five-*barrio* area in Cali. It was pointed out in that chapter that the level of resources available to the Cali area includes a number of special programs not available elsewhere and that the three-quarters resource level more closely models the relative resource scarcity faced by the communities intended to be described by the child mortality project. In a later section we consider the effect of both increasing and decreasing resources from the reference $0.75R$ level.

After trying several initial starting points (a starting point consists of a set of initial activity levels), several slightly different solutions were obtained. The highest of these consistently exhausted registered nurse time but stopped short of exhausting either the total budget or the supplies budget because of the small size of the increase in the number of survivors (NOS) with increases in the activities requiring pesos but not nursing time. By restricting the search to activities not using registered nurses, the intermediate solution became an initial starting point for a second level optimization using a smaller stopping criteria (ε), which led to still further improvements in NOS and the exhaustion of both registered nurse time and the available budget for supplies. Morbidity, case fatality, and mortality rates that result from this solution are given in Table 8–1. The activity levels, expressed as a percentage of the applicable demographic or epidemiological groups, are listed on the right-hand side of Table 8–2. Alternatively, expressed in terms of interventions used by the target groups, the solution is listed on the left in Table 8–2.

With the optimum allocation of resources, the neonatal mortality rate falls to 22/1000 births, the infant mortality rate falls to 42/1000, and the early childhood rate is 20/1000. The number of survivors is 11,702. A large

Table 8–1. Morbidity and Mortality Rates with Optimum Resource Allocation (resources = 0.75R).

	0–1 Month Age Group	1–12 Month Age Group	12–60 Month Age Group
I. Marginal morbidity rates			
Low birth weight	.044		
Infection	.074		
Birth trauma	.034		
Tetanus	.000		
Malnutrition		.023	.025
Diarrhea		.048	.039
Respiratory		.039	.010
Immunizable		.003	.002
II. Fatality rates			
Tetanus, all states	.875		
Low birth weight only	.130		
Birth trauma only	.202		
Infection only	.019		
Low birth weight & birth trauma	.293		
Low birth weight & infection	.223		
Birth trauma & infection	.237		
Low birth weight & birth trauma & infection	.336		
Malnutrition only		.0036	.0014
Diarrhea only		.0022	.0007
Respiratory only		.0065	.0012
Immunizable only		.0577	.0185
Malnutrition & immunizable		.1109	.0333
Malnutrition & diarrhea		.0110	.0037
Malnutrition & respiratory		.0156	.0036
Other combinations		.0346	.0135
III. Age group mortality rate	.022	.020	.020
Number of survivors			11819

part of the reduction in mortality as compared with the baseline simulation in Chapter 7 comes from the large decrease in morbidity for diarrhea and malnutrition. Mortality is also decreased by lower case fatality rates. The reduction in malnutrition has an important effect of shifting remaining morbidity into joint disease categories with lower fatality rates. In addition, the reduction in morbidity makes it feasible to treat essentially all morbidity using outpatient care. This leads to still further reduction in the fatality rates.

As expected from the simulations in Chapter 7, the promotora and mass media activities play a central role in motivating the use of other health activities and in encouraging breast feeding and early prenatal care. In

Table 8–2. Optimum Intervention and Activity Levels with Resources = 0.75R.

	Intervention	I_i		Activity	X_i	
	PROMOTER	1	.90	PROMOTER	1	.90
	AWTXINF	2		AWEXAM	2	
EXAM &	AFEDETX	3		PWEXAM	3	.76
	AWTXANE	4	.67	AWTXINF	4	
EXAM &	PWTXINF 2	5	.04	AWTXANE	5	.67
	PWNUTLBW 2	6	.04	AFEDEFTX	6	
	PWETEIMM 2	7	.05	PWTXINF	7	.74
	PWHCED 2	8	.01	PWNUTLBW	8	.75
	PWNUT 2	9	.04	PWTETIMM	9	.97
	DELINLBW	10		PWHCED	10	.20
EXAM & (WITH EARLY CARE)	PWTXINF 1	11	.70	PWNUT	11	.76
	PWNUTLBW 1	12	.70	DELIN	12	
	PWTETIMM 1	13	.88	DELMW	13	.64
	PWHCED 1	14	.18	DELPROM	14	.26
	PWNUT 1	15	.71	DELINLBW	15	
	DELIN	16		1OUTP	16	1.00
	DELMW	17	.57	1 INP	17	
	DELPROM	18	.23	H2OHOME	18	.30
	BF	19	.78	H2OWALK	19	.70
	H2OHOME	20	.30	TOILET	20	.13
	H2OWALK	21	.70	LATRINE	21	.87
	TOILET	22	.13	MMEDIA	22	1.00
	LATRINE	23	.87	IMMDPTPM	23	.50
	MMEDIA	24	.99	2 WBD	24	.96
	1 OUTP	25	.98	2 NUTCH	25	.45
	1 INP	26		2 NUTBF	26	
	IMMDPTPM	27	.50	2 OUTP	27	1.00
	2 WBC	28	.91	2 INP	28	
	2 NUTCH	29	.45	3 WBC	29	.78
	2 BFWSUP	30		3 NUTCH	30	.60
	2 BFNOSUP	31	.78	3 OUTP	30	1.00
	2 OUTP	32	.99	3 INP	32	
	2 INP	33				
	3 WBC	34	.78			
	3 NUTCH	35	.60			
	3 OUTP	36	.98			
	3 INP	37				

spite of the fact that examinations, treatment, nutritional programs, and tetanus immunization for pregnant women are some of the more costly (see Table 6–14) alternatives considered, these activities are selected at high participation levels, especially in combination with early detection of pregnancy.

High activity levels were also found for water activities and latrines. Experiments with the model revealed that, at the given levels for the other activities, the marginal cost effectiveness of H2OHOME and H2OWALK are not distinctly different, and in the first level optimization the solution covered 60 percent of all households with the percentage split about equally between the two activities. On the other hand latrines, while less than one-third to one-half as effective as toilets, are only one-twentieth of the cost. For both water and sanitation, the second level optimization produces 100-percent coverage of all households by these activities.

Under the optimal solution, immunizations would cover only 50 percent of children. Compared to other activities in the optimum activity set, immunization is expensive and, since morbidity rates for immunizable diseases are low, must cover a broad demographic base to achieve significant reductions in mortality. Caution should be used in assessing this result, however, since the immunization cost data were obtained from a separately administered program and appeared to be more complete and accurate than the clinical and nutritional cost data. Impact coefficients for immunization data are also better established and not based on subjective estimates. Thus, in spite of the optimal solution, a reasonable strategy might include a higher activity level for immunizations because their effectiveness is predicted with more confidence than for other activities.

Nutritional activities for infants are not selected as cost effective. The marked reduction in malnutrition in the infant age group is achieved through breast feeding and nutritional counseling in the well-baby clinic and by the promotora. A significant part of the reduction is also achieved through the reduction in diarrhea and the interrelationship between diarrhea and malnutrition.

OPTIMUM RESOURCE ALLOCATION AND THE LEVEL OF RESOURCES

An interesting question centers on how the pattern of resource allocation changes as the quantity of all resources increased. To examine this question, we consider the optimum activity levels as the availability of all resources—peso budgets, medical doctor and nursing time, and facilities—goes from 25 percent to 125 percent of the levels tallied for the Cali community. Results for the alternative optimizations are reported in Table 8–3. To simplify interpretation and to emphasize the difference between prenatal programs with and without early detection of pregnancy, the optimum outcomes are reported in terms of intervention coverage rather than activities.

The interventions selected for a resource-poor community ($0.25R$) are promotion, breast feeding, latrines, water, well-baby clinics, tetanus, immunization, iron fortification tablets, and outpatient services for children in the first twenty-eight days. An examination of the unit resource

Table 8–3. Comparison of Results from Alternative Optimizations.

	Intervention	I_i	Resource Level				
			.25R	*.5R*	*.75R*	*1.00R*	*1.25R*
	PROMOTER	1	.85	.98	.90	.89	.89
	AWTXINF	2				.12	.22
EXAM &	AFEDEFTX	3	.02	.17		.11	.22
	AWTXANE	4	.47	.50	.67	.71	.71
	PWTXINF 2	5			.04	.04	.05
	PWNUTLBW 2	6			.04	.04	.05
EXAM &	PWETEIMM 2	7	.02	.06	.05	.06	.06
	PWHCED 2	8			.01	.04	.05
	PWNUT 2	9			.04	.04	.05
	DELINLBW	10				.28	.31
	PWTXINF 1	11			.70	.66	.80
EXAM &	PWNUTLBW 1	12			.70	.60	.71
(WITH	PWTETIMM 1	13	.18	.84	.88	.88	.88
EARLY	PWHCED 1	14			.18	.58	.72
CARE)	PWNUT 1	15			.71	.62	.76
	DELIN	16					
	DELMW	17		.10	.57	.33	.47
	DELPROM	18		.41	.23	.38	.35
	BF	19	.73	.78	.78	.78	.78
	H2OHOME	20	.13	.32	.30	.78	.73
	H2OWALK	21	.23	.29	.70	.27	.27
	TOILET	22		.12	.13	.38	.44
	LATRINE	23	.99	.88	.87	.44	.44
	MMEDIA	24	.72	.78	.99	.99	1.00
	1 OUTP	25	.26	.94	.98		
	1 INP	26				.97	.99
	IMMDPTPM	27		.01	.50	.93	1.00
	2 WBC	28	.52	.90	.91	.91	.91
	2 NUTCH	29			.45	.10	.11
	2 BFWSUP	30					
	2 BFNOSUP	31	.73	.78	.78	.78	.78
	2 OUTP	32	.01	.99	.99	.80	.07
	2 INP	33				.20	.92
	3 WBC	34	.77	.82	.78	.77	.77
	3 NUTCH	35	.17	.47	.60	.48	.47
	3 OUTP	36		.42	.98	.98	.97
	3 INP	37					.01
	Age group mortality rates						
	0–1		.035	.030	.022	.016	.015
	1–12		.040	.022	.020	.017	.015
	12–60		.039	.026	.020	.019	.019
	Number of survivors		11106	11507	11702	11819	11863

costs (Table 6–14) reveals that, except for tetanus immunization, outpatient clinic facilities, and water services, these activities are low in cost. Also, the base population (see Table 6–16), and, therefore, the total number of units needed, is relatively small for tetanus immunization and outpatient services.

As resources increase to 0.5*R* the level of the activities selected under 0.25*R* increases and promotora visits after delivery (DELPROM), outpatient care (OUTP), and a nutritional program for children 12–60 (3NUTCH) are added. An effect of the promotora visit after delivery is to identify neonatal morbidity conditions. This activity works in conjunction with the expanded use of neonatal outpatient care to reduce fatality rates. With the resource level at 0.25*R*, breast feeding provides a large decrease in malnutrition in the infant age group and the rate for the 12–60 group is lowered to 0.05 by the indirect effects of promotora, latrines, and water. With the increase in available resources to 0.5*R* the nutritional program for children in the 12–60 age group is selected and the rate of malnutrition in this age group falls still further to 0.03.

Optimum allocations above 0.75*R* include the addition of higher cost activities, especially immunizations, institutional delivery of low-birth-weight-risk mothers, and inpatient care for the first two age groups. A notable feature of the change in allocations above 0.75*R* is an upgrading of alternative activities. Boundary conditions in the computer program restrict the sum of all delivery activities to be less than or equal to the total number of births, the sum of all inpatient and outpatient treatments to be less than or equal to the number of cases of morbidity, and the sum of water and sanitation alternatives to be less than or equal to the number of households. As resources increase, there is an upgrading of services within these boundaries—toilets replace latrines, water in home replaces public fountains, midwife and institutional deliveries replace unattended deliveries, and inpatient care replaces outpatient care.

The payoff from upgrading becomes successively less, however, as resource levels increase. Figure 8–4 shows the tapering off of the number of survivors as resource availability increases. Shown somewhat differently, Figure 8–5 reveals the rapidly diminishing returns to changes in *R*. In interpeting this diagram it should be noted that although the percentage change in NOS is small the percentage change in the mortality rate may be large. Thus, an increase in resources from 1.00*R* to 1.25*R* increases the number of survivors by only 0.04 percent but decreases the mortality rate by nearly 10 percent.

A second caution is not to interpret Figure 8–5 as indicating that rapidly diminishing returns necessarily start between 0.75*R* and 1.0*R*. Experiments demonstrate that the shape of the curve is sensitive to the size of the responses on the morbidity survey. The reported results are based on the

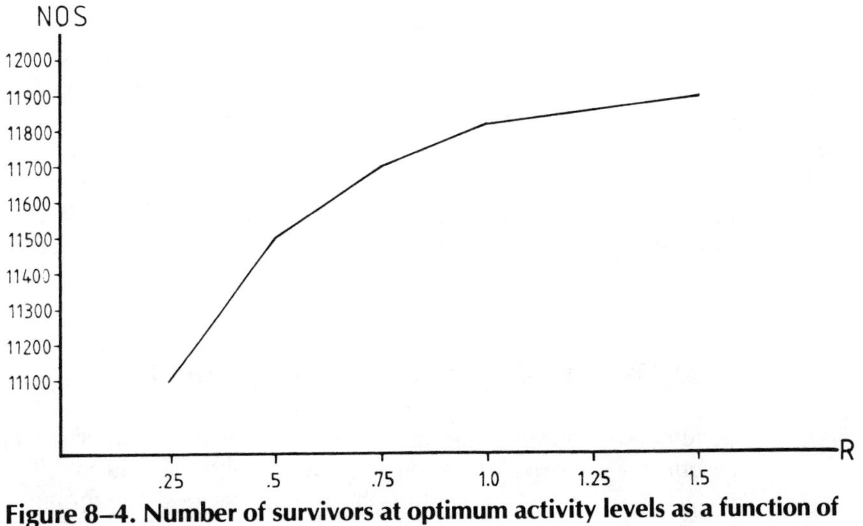

Figure 8–4. Number of survivors at optimum activity levels as a function of resource level.

unaltered average survey responses. If, as may be psychologically plausible, the respondents uniformly overestimated the impacts of the alternative activities, the true coefficients would be much lower, although the relative emphasis on alternative activities would not change. In a sensitivity test using responses diminished by a constant proportion, the point of rapidly diminishing returns comes at higher resource levels.

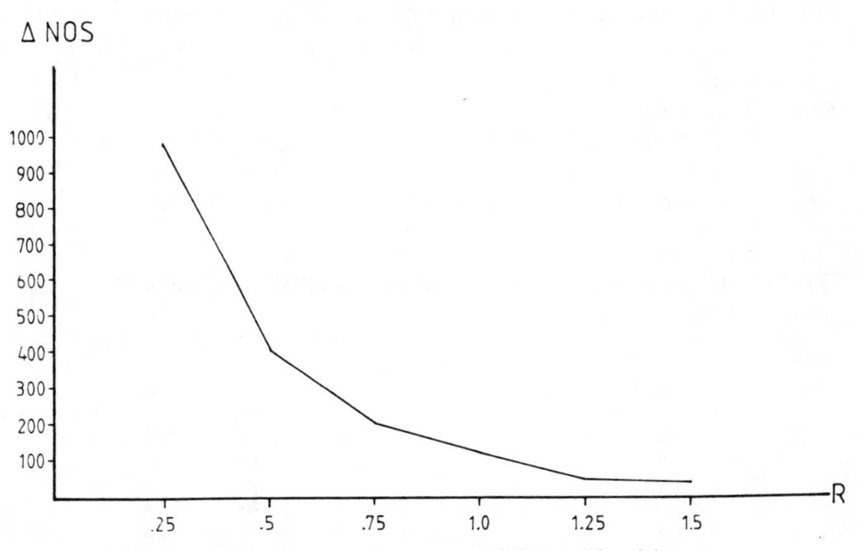

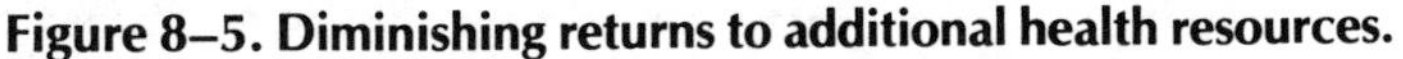
Figure 8–5. Diminishing returns to additional health resources.

Considering these cautionary observations, the response of the number of survivors to increases in the level of health resources does not imply that further investment in this sector should cease after 1.5R or some other given resource level, but it does imply that the dramatic decreases in mortality come at fairly low resource levels through health promotion, education, water and sanitation, breast feeding, and tetanus immunization. At higher resource levels, the payoff to additional health resources is not as dramatic and should be compared carefully with other priority areas competing for the use of community resources.

SHADOW VALUE OF ADDITIONAL RESOURCES

Seven resource categories are included in the allocation problem. Not all resource categories are exhausted at the optimal solution. The proportion of available resources in each category used at the optimum activity levels as the general availability of resources goes from 0.25R to 1.25R is reported in Table 8–4. The constraining resources at all levels are registered nurse time and either the supplies budget or the total budget. Hospital beds, medical doctor time, and institutional facilities remain far below constraining levels and only come in to use as the level of all community resources becomes larger and an upgrading of services becomes involved in the optimal solution. To some extent, the level of medical doctor time and institutional resources may be unrealistically high because of the presence in the baseline community of a teaching hospital, although an effort was made to correct for this problem in tallying the available resources. But even making allowances for the possibility of such an overestimate, it is apparent that at low resource levels the important constraints are peso funds and nursing time.

An indication of the importance of the two binding constraints can be obtained by estimating the increase in the number of survivors with a relaxation in these constraints. That is, we compute the "shadow" values of

Table 8–4. Proportion of Total Resources Used at Optimum Levels of Activities.

Resources Available	*Total Budget*	*Supplies Budget*	*MD Time*	*RN Time*	*AN Time*	*Bed Days*	*Capital Capacity*
0.25R	.90	1.00	.16	1.00	.63	.00	.02
0.50R	.97	1.00	.22	1.00	.84	.00	.01
0.75R	.88	1.00	.23	1.00	.90	.00	.01
1.00R	1.00	.99	.39	1.00	.68	.40	.04
1.25R	1.00	.99	.58	1.00	.72	.84	.07

the constraints by calculating the change in NOS with an increase in, alternatively, the supplies budget and auxiliary nurse time. At the 0.25*R* resource level, the shadow value of an increase in the supplies budget of 10,000 pesos is an increase of 1.5 survivors. At the 0.75 resource level, the shadow value of 10,000 pesos is an increase of 0.6 in the number of survivors. The decline in the shadow value is expected given the generally diminishing returns to program size demonstrated by the simulations in Chapter 7. Measured in terms of pesos per additional life saved, the shadow value is 6667 pesos ($195 US) at the lower resource level and 16,667 pesos ($476 US) at the higher level.

Looking at the value of additional registered nurse time, it is found that an additional sixty minutes (per twenty-eight-day period) will increase the number of survivors by 0.9 when the general resource level is 0.25*R* and by 0.6 when the general resource level is 0.75*R*. Shadow values have implications for planning. With regard to nursing time, the shadow values indicate that the training of registered nurses should be an important component of manpower planning, perhaps receiving some of the resources that are now going to physician training.

It is difficult to compare shadow values to obtain an indication of the relative importance of the binding constraints since one is measured in time and the other pesos. A simple conversion of registered nurse time to equivalent peso value, or vice versa, is not feasible because, on the one hand, there are bottlenecks in the training of nurses that are not reflected in the wage, and, on the other hand, there are practical and political restrictions on the expansion of public budgets that are not reflected in the face monetary value of the budgets. Some indication of the relative importance of the constraints is given, however, by the behavior of the optimization program. At the lower general resource levels (0.25*R*–0.75*R*), registered nurse time is exhausted in the first level optimization with the larger stoping criterion (ε) and is therefore a more binding constraint than the peso budgets, which were exhausted only with the second level optimization and finer stopping criterion. For both constraints the shadow values demonstrate the large payoff, in terms of reduced child mortality, that would accompany relatively small increases in the constraining resources.

SUMMARY

A nonlinear optimization program is used to find the allocation of resources that maximizes the number of children who survive to an age of sixty months. The child mortality model is sufficiently complicated that the true optimum may not be discovered, but the optimum suggested by the program is probably capable of only a small improvement without policy significance. A greater restriction on the application of the results is the experimental nature of the survey process used to generate the impact coefficients and the imprecise data available for costs. Both of these factors dictate that the optimization results be given only a qualitative interpretation.

Using general levels of resources that vary from 0.25 to 1.25 of the baseline level of resources in the Cali community, it is found that sharp reductions in mortality come from reducing the incidence of diarrhea, low birth weight, and malnutrition. At low levels of resources, the activities selected for emphasis are health promotion, water and sanitation, and well-baby clinics. These activities act to promote breast feeding and to lower diarrhea and, through disease interaction, to lower malnutrition. Outpatient treatment for neonatal children and prenatal tetanus immunization are also chosen for resource-poor communities.

As the community resources increase to middle levels, nutritional activities, immunizations, and outpatient care for the older age groups are adopted. Prenatal care activities and the general coverage of the programs selected at the lower resource levels are also increased. At the highest resource levels considered, an upgrading of activities occurs as inpatient care replaces outpatient care and home water and toilets replace public fountains and latrines.

The reduction in child mortality with the optimum use of resources is dramatic at low resource levels and diminishes as resources become more abundant. Similarly, the value of the constraining resources falls as the general level of resources increases. Registered nurse time and the peso budgets are found to be the binding constraints, and a high proportion of available auxiliary nurse time is used in most of the optimization experiments. A possible implication is that manpower training programs should place more emphasis on the training of nurses.

NOTE

1. The optimization technique is discussed in detail in D. L. Keefer and B. S. Gottfried, "Differential Constraint Scaling in Penalty Function Optimization," *American Institute of Industrial Engineers Transactions* 2 (1970): 281–289. Also see R. Fletcher and M. J. D. Powell, "A Rapidly Convergent Descent Method for Minimization," *Computer Journal* 6 (1962–1963): 163–168.

Appendix

The Child Mortality Model FORTRAN Simulation Program

This appendix lists the computer program used for the simulation of the patterns of child morbidity and mortality discussed in Chapter 7. The program is comprised of a main program (MAIN) and five subprograms (INIT, BOUND, PCALC, PHCOM, PHVFIN). MAIN reads in the test levels of the activities (X vector) and calls INIT to read in the morbidity, fatality, and usage coefficients; BOUND to check the resource and epidemiological constraints; and PCALC to calculate the morbidity and mortality rates. PCALC also calls PHCOM and PHVFIN to compute the joint disease state probabilities. The programs are a direct translation into fortran code of the model set forth in the text. With minor modifications—the omission of MAIN and all write statements—the simulation program becomes the subprogram used to calculate the objective (number of survivors) maximized by the optimization program.

MAIN PROGRAM

```
   1              DIMENSION X(32),T(32,11),G(60)
   2              DOUBLE PRECISION X,T,G,Y
   3              DATA G/60*0.0/
   4              CALL INIT
   5              READ(3,100)M
   6              DO 6 I=1,M
   7              READ(3,101) (T(J,I),J=1,32)
   8          6   CONTINUE
   9              DO 10 K=1,M
  10              DO 20 L=1,32
  11              X(L)=T(L,K)
  12         20   CONTINUE
  13              WRITE(2,102)K
  14              WRITE(2,103)X
  15              CALL BOUND(X,G)
  16              CALL PCALC(X,Y)
  17         10   CONTINUE
  18        100   FORMAT(I3)
  19        101   FORMAT(12F6.0/12F6.0/8F6.0)
  20        102   FORMAT('1','INTERVENTION LEVELS SET #',I2)
  21        103   FORMAT('0','X  :',12F6.0/' ',4X,12F6.0/' ',4X,8F6.0)
  22              STOP
  23              END
END OF FILE
```

```
1           SUBROUTINE INIT
2           DIMENSION S(6),SU(5,3),SUC(2,5,3),SZ(4,3),SZC(6,4,3)
3           DIMENSION N(12),IUC(2,5,3),IZC(37,4,3),IGC(3,8,3)
4           DIMENSION MBC(4,4,3),MCC(2),PHU(4,3),PHL(4,3),MAC(4,3)
5           DIMENSION MOK(3),R(7),RUA(7,32),PART(18)
6     C
7           DOUBLE PRECISION S,SU,SUC,SZ,SZC,N,IUC,IZC,IGC,MAC,MBC,MCC
8           DOUBLE PRECISION PHU,PHL,MOK,F12,R,RUA,Z2,Z3,Z4,Z5
9     C
10          INTEGER HAG,HD,NN,HS,HU,HZ,NZZ,HR,HIU,HIZ,HIG,MX,PART
11    C
12          COMMON /SEC1/ N,R,RUA
13          COMMON /SEC2/ MBC,PHU,PHL,SU,SZ,IUC,IZC,IGC,MAC,MCC,MOK,F12
14    C
15    C IDENTIFY SURVEY SET(S) USED.
16    C
17          NP=1
18          READ(1,100)PART(1)
19          IF(PART(1).EQ.99)READ(1,100)NP,(PART(I),I=1,NP)
20          WRITE(2,200)(PART(I),I=1,NP)
21    C
22    C READ IN ARRAY DIMENSIONS, THIS RUN (.LE.DECLARED DIMENSIONS).
23    C
24          READ(3,100)HAG,HD,NN,HS,HU,HZ,NZZ,HR,HIU,HIZ,HIG,MX
25    C
26    C SET RESOURCE CONSTRAINTS AND "# OF UNITS OF RESOURCE J REQUIRED PER
27    C UNIT OF ACTIVITY I" INFO.
28    C
29          READ(3,102)(R(I),I=1,HR)
30          READ(3,103)((RUA(J,I),J=1,HR),I=1,MX)
31    C
32    C READ CONSTANT VECTORS FOR U, Z, AND G. THEN READ SES DATA AND COMPUTE
33    C SES FACTORS FOR THE RUN.
34    C
35          READ(1,101)((SU(J,I),J=1,HU),I=1,HAG)
36          READ(1,101)((SZ(J,I),J=1,HZ),I=1,HAG)
37    C
38          READ(1,101)(S(I),I=1,HS)
39          READ(1,101)(((SUC(K,J,I),K=1,2),J=1,HU),I=1,HAG)
40          READ(1,101)(((SZC(K,J,I),K=1,HS),J=1,HZ),I=1,HAG)
41    C
42          DO 16 K=1,2
43          DO 14 I=1,3
44          DO 12 J=1,2
45          SU(J,I)=SU(J,I)+SUC(K,J,I)*S(K)
46       12 CONTINUE
47       14 CONTINUE
48          SU(3,1)=SU(3,1)+SUC(K,3,1)*S(K)
49          SU(4,1)=SU(4,1)+SUC(K,4,1)*S(K)
50          SU(5,1)=SU(5,1)+SUC(K,5,1)*S(K)
51       16 CONTINUE
52    C
53          DO 22 I=1,3
54          SZ(1,I)=SZ(1,I)+SZC(2,1,I)*S(2)+SZC(3,1,I)*S(3)
55          SZ(2,I)=SZ(2,I)+SZC(2,2,I)*S(2)+SZC(4,2,I)*S(4)
56       22 CONTINUE
57          DO 26 I=2,3
58          DO 24 J=3,4
59          SZ(J,I)=SZ(J,I)+SZC(4,J,I)*S(4)
```

```
 60        24   CONTINUE
 61        26   CONTINUE
 62             DO 34 J=1,3,2
 63             DO 32 K=5,6
 64             SZ(J,1)=SZ(J,1)+SZC(K,J,1)*S(K)
 65        32   CONTINUE
 66        34   CONTINUE
 67             SZ(2,1)=SZ(2,1)+SZC(3,2,1)*S(3)
 68       C
 69       C INITIALIZE REMAINING COEFFICIENT AND PARAMETER ARRAYS.
 70       C FIRST, INTERVENTION COEF'S AND PHIS 'UPPER' & LOWER BOUNDS.
 71       C
 72             READ(1,101) (((IUC(K,J,I),K=1,HIU),J=1,HU),I=1,HAG)
 73             READ(1,101) (((IZC(K,J,I),K=1,HIZ),J=1,HZ),I=1,HAG)
 74             READ(1,101) (((IGC(K,J,I),K=1,HIG),J=1,HD),I=1,HAG)
 75             READ(1,101) ((PHU(J,I),J=1,HZ),I=1,HAG)
 76             READ(1,101) ((PHL(J,I),J=1,HZ),I=1,HAG)
 77             IZC(7,4,1)=.6
 78             IZC(13,4,1)=.95
 79       C
 80       C THEN POP STRATA AND MORTALITY RATE CONSTANTS.
 81       C
 82             READ(3,104) (N(I),I=1,NN)
 83             READ(3,106) (MOK(I),I=1,HAG)
 84       C
 85       C LASTLY, WEIGHT 'A' ON PHIS, INTERACTIVE COEF'S & LAGGED FACTORS.
 86       C
 87             READ(1,101) ((MAC(J,I),J=1,HZ),I=1,HAG)
 88             READ(1,101) (((MBC(K,J,I),K=1,HZ),J=1,HZ),I=1,HAG)
 89             READ(1,101) (MCC(I),I=1,NZZ)
 90       C
 91       C COMPUTE (FOR THE RUN) THE FACTOR NEEDED FOR SOLVING THE SYSTEM OF
 92       C SIMULTANEOUS EQUATIONS THAT OCCURS IN EVERY PASS THRU PH A.G. 2
 93       C SOLUTION CODE.
 94       C
 95             F12=1.0/(1.0-MBC(1,2,2)*MBC(2,1,2)-MBC(1,3,2)*MBC(3,1,2))
 96       C
 97       C WRITE OUT SAMPLE OF SES DATA AND THEN HEADING FOR PCALC OUTPUT.
 98       C THESE STATEMENTS ARE OMITTED IN OPTIMIZATION RUNS.
 99       C
100             WRITE(2,202)S(3),S(4),SU(1,1)
101             WRITE(2,203)SZ(2,2),MOK(3)
102             WRITE(2,206)R
103             WRITE(2,207)N
104             WRITE(2,204)
105             WRITE(2,205)
106       C
107       100   FORMAT(20I3)
108       101   FORMAT(9F10.6)
109       102   FORMAT(7F10.0)
110       103   FORMAT(7F10.3)
111       104   FORMAT(9F8.0)
112       106   FORMAT(9F8.5)
113       200   FORMAT('-','THIS RUN USES SURVEY DATA SUPPLIED BY PARTICIPANT(S)',
114            116I3)
115       202   FORMAT('0','S(3)=',F8.4,' S(4)=',F8.4,' SU(1,1)=',F8.4)
116       203   FORMAT(' ','SZ(2,2)=',F8.4,' MOK(3)=',F8.5)
117       204   FORMAT('-','FOR THE SPECIFIED SET X OF INTERVENTION LEVELS, THE AS
118            1SOCIATED SETS OF CONSTRAINT CHECKS AND MORBIDITY,')
119       205   FORMAT(' ','INTERSECTIONAL, FATALITY, & MORTALITY RATES ARE LISTED
```

```
   120            1 AND THEN THE NUMBER OF SURVIVORS, NOS :')
   121        206  FORMAT('-','R :',7F10.0)
   122        207  FORMAT(' ','N :',12F8.0)
   123             RETURN
   124             END
END OF FILE
```

```
     1            SUBROUTINE BOUND(X,G)
     2      C
     3            DIMENSION X(32),G(24),N(12),R(7),RUA(7,32)
     4      C
     5            DOUBLE PRECISION X,G,N,R,RUA,XMAX25,XMAX30
     6      C
     7            COMMON/SEC1/N,R,RUA
     8      C
     9            DATA XMAX25/2840.0/,XMAX30/12075.0/
    10      C
    11      C FIRST CHECK RESOURCE CONSTRAINTS.
    12      C
    13            DO 12 K=1,7
    14            G(K)=0.0
    15            DO 10 J=1,32
    16            G(K)=G(K)+RUA(K,J)*X(J)
    17         10 CONTINUE
    18            G(K)=G(K)-R(K)
    19         12 CONTINUE
    20      C
    21      C FINALLY SEE TO THE "ADDITIONAL RESTRICTIONS".
    22      C
    23            G(8)=X(4)-N(4)*X(2)/N(2)
    24            G(9)=X(5)-N(2)*X(1)/N(1)
    25            G(10)=X(6)-N(5)*X(2)/N(2)
    26            G(11)=X(7)-N(6)*X(3)/N(3)
    27            G(12)=X(8)-N(7)*X(3)/N(3)
    28            G(13)=X(10)-X(3)
    29            G(14)=X(11)-X(3)
    30            G(15)=X(12)+X(13)+X(14)+X(15)-N(8)
    31            G(16)=X(15)-N(9)*X(3)/N(3)
    32            G(17)=X(18)+X(19)-N(1)
    33            G(18)=X(20)+X(21)-N(1)
    34            G(19)=X(5)+X(6)-N(2)
    35            G(20)=X(16)+X(17)-N(10)
    36            G(21)=X(27)+X(28)-N(11)
    37            G(22)=X(31)+X(32)-N(12)
    38            G(23)=X(25)-XMAX25*X(1)/N(1)
    39            G(24)=X(30)-XMAX30*X(1)/N(1)
    40      C
    41      C OUTPUT
    42      C
    43            WRITE(2,101)
    44            WRITE(2,102)G
    45        101 FORMAT('0','G (G(I).LE.0 = CONSTRAINT I HAS BEEN MET) :')
    46        102 FORMAT(' ',5F11.1)
    47            RETURN
    48            END
END OF FILE
```

```
1          SUBROUTINE PCALC(X,NOS)
2    C
3          DIMENSION X(32),SU(5,3),SZ(4,3),N(12),IUC(2,5,3)
4          DIMENSION IZC(37,4,3),IGC(3,8,3),MAC(4,3),MBC(4,4,3)
5          DIMENSION PHL(4,3),MOK(3),XP(32),IN(37)
6          DIMENSION U(5),Y(5),Z(4),AZ(4),PH(4),PHV(8),PD(8)
7          DIMENSION MCC(2),PHU(4,3),DX1(15)
8    C
9          DOUBLE PRECISION X,NOS,SU,SZ,N,IUC,IZC,MAC,MBC,MCC,PHU,PHL
10         DOUBLE PRECISION AZ,MOK,XP,TXP,MO1,IN,U,Y,Z,PH,PHV,PD,F12
11         DOUBLE PRECISION F13,D1,D2,T1,T2,MO,N32,N33,PHVSUM,WT,DMIN1
12         DOUBLE PRECISION DMAX1,DEXP,PL11,PL12,IGC,MOFIN,NOSUB
13   C
14         INTEGER DX1
15   C
16         DATA XP/32*0.0/,NOSUB/12461.46/
17         DATA Z/4*0.0/,IN/37*0.0/
18         DATA DX1/1,2,3,4,2,5,5,7,3,3,3,8,8,8,9/
19   C
20         COMMON /SEC1/ N
21         COMMON /SEC2/ MBC,PHU,PHL,SU,SZ,IUC,IZC,IGC,MAC,MCC,MOK,F12
22         COMMON /SEC3/ PH,PHV
23   C
24   C FOR EACH AGE GROUP IN TURN, 0-1 THEN 1-12 THEN 12-60, THE FOLLOWING 5
25   C SECTIONS ARE COMPLETED:
26   C  SECTION 1: GET TEST INTERVENTION LEVELS.
27   C    STEP 1.1: CONVERT CHOSEN INTERVENTION LEVELS, X, TO PER CAPITA (OF
28   C              RELEVANT  POPULATION) LEVELS, XP.
29   C    STEP 1.2: COMPUTE USAGE DEMAND, FOR CLASSES OF INTERVENTIONS.
30   C    STEP 1.3: CONVERT U TO PERCENTAGE USAGE DEMAND, Y.
31   C    STEP 1.4: WHERE USAGE CHECKS ARE SPECIFIED, SET TEST LEVELS, IN, TO
32   C              MINIMUM OF XP & Y, OTHERWISE USE XP.
33   C  SECTION 2: CALCULATE PH.
34   C    STEP 2.1: COMPUTE Z.
35   C    STEP 2.2: CALCULATE AZ USING LOGIT FUNCTION.
36   C    STEP 2.3: CALCULATE PH
37   C  SECTION 3: FIND PHV.
38   C    STEP 3.1: CALL PHCOM FOR PT,PA,P2,P3,AND HENCE PHV.
39   C  SECTION 4: COMPUTE PD.
40   C    STEP 4.1: PERFORM ADDITIONAL CONVERSIONS,X TO XP, USING PHV RESULTS.
41   C    STEP 4.2: DO CORRESPONDING ADDITIONAL XP/Y COMPARISON CHECKS TO GET
42   C              MINIMUM IN LEVEL
43   C    STEP 4.3: NOW GENERATE PD FUNCTION.
44   C  SECTION 5: GET THE AGE GROUP'S MORTALITY RATE, MO.
45   C
46   C THE OPTIMIZATION OBJECTIVE , NOS (# OF SURVIVORS AT THE END OF
47   C 60 MOS), IS THEN FIGURED AS A FUNCTION OF THE 12-60 A.G.'S BASELINE
48   C POPULATION, N33, AND ITS MO.
49   C
50   C SO ON WITH THE CODE.
51   C
52   C AGE GROUP 0-1
53   C  SECTION 1
54   C   STEP 1.1
55   C
56         WRITE(2,202)
57         DO 10 K=1,15
58         L=DX1(K)
59         XP(K)=X(K)/N(L)
```

```
 60        10  CONTINUE
 61            DO 12 K=18,22
 62            XP(K)=X(K)/N(1)
 63        12  CONTINUE
 64      C
 65      C   STEP 1.2 & STEP 1.3
 66      C
 67            DO 14 K=1,5
 68            U(K)=SU(K,1)+IUC(1,K,1)*XP(1)+IUC(2,K,1)*XP(22)
 69            Y(K)=1.0/(1.0+DEXP(-U(K)))
 70        14  CONTINUE
 71      C
 72      C   STEP 1.4
 73      C
 74            IN(2)=DMIN1(XP(4),Y(1))
 75            IN(3)=DMIN1(XP(6),Y(1))
 76            IN(4)=DMIN1(XP(5),Y(1))
 77            TXP=(X(12)+X(13)+X(14)+X(15))/N(8)
 78            T1=DMIN1(TXP,Y(2))
 79            IN(10)=T1*XP(15)
 80            IN(16)=T1*XP(12)
 81            IN(17)=T1*XP(13)
 82            IN(18)=T1*XP(14)
 83            Y(3)=T1+(1.0-T1)*Y(3)
 84            IN(1)=XP(1)
 85            IN(19)=Y(4)
 86            IN(20)=XP(18)
 87            IN(21)=XP(19)
 88            IN(22)=XP(20)
 89            IN(23)=XP(21)
 90            IN(24)=XP(22)
 91            DO 21 K1=5,9
 92            K2=K1+6
 93            J=K1+2
 94            T1=DMIN1(XP(J),Y(2))
 95            IN(K2)=Y(5)*T1
 96            IN(K1)=(1-Y(5))*T1
 97        21  CONTINUE
 98      C
 99      C  SECTION 2
100      C   STEP 2.1
101      C
102            DO 23 K=1,2
103            Z(K)=SZ(K,1)
104            DO 26 I=1,24
105            Z(K)=Z(K)+IZC(I,K,1)*IN(I)
106        26  CONTINUE
107        23  CONTINUE
108            Z(2)=Z(2)+IZC(16,2,1)*IN(10)
109            Z(3)=SZ(3,1)+IZC(5,3,1)*IN(5)+IZC(10,3,1)*IN(10)+IZC(11,
110           13,1)*IN(11)+IZC(16,3,1)*IN(16)+IZC(17,3,1)*IN(17)
111            Z(4)=IZC(1,4,1)*IN(1)+IZC(8,4,1)*IN(8)+IZC(14,4,1)*IN(14
112           1)+IZC(16,4,1)*IN(16)+IZC(17,4,1)*IN(17)+IZC(18,4,1)*IN(18)
113            Z(4)=Z(4)+IZC(16,4,1)*IN(10)+SZ(4,1)
114      C
115      C   STEP 2.2
116      C
117            DO 37 K=1,4
118            AZ(K)=MAC(K,1)*(PHU(K,1)/(1+DEXP(-Z(K)))+PHL(K,1))
119        37  CONTINUE
```

```
120      C
121      C   STEP 2.3
122      C
123            PH(1)=AZ(1)
124            PH(2)=AZ(2)+MBC(1,2,1)*PH(1)
125            PH(3)=AZ(3)
126      C
127      C    ADJUST PH4 FOR TETANUS INOCULATION LEVEL DOMINANCE.
128      C
129            PH(4)=(1-IZC(7,4,1)*IN(7)-IZC(13,4,1)*IN(13))*AZ(4)
130      C  SECTION 3
131      C   STEP 3.1
132      C
133            CALL PHCOM1
134      C
135      C  SECTION 4
136      C   STEP 4.1
137      C
138            PHVSUM=0.0
139            DO 39 K=1,8
140            PHVSUM=PHVSUM+PHV(K)
141         39 CONTINUE
142            WT=N(8)*PHVSUM
143            XP(16)=X(16)/WT
144            XP(17)=X(17)/WT
145            TXP=XP(16)+XP(17)
146      C
147      C   STEP 4.2
148      C
149            T2=DMIN1(TXP,Y(3))
150            T1=1-T2
151            IN(26)=DMIN1(XP(17),T2)
152            IN(25)=T2-IN(26)
153      C
154      C   STEP 4.3
155      C
156            DO 48 K=1,8
157            PD(K)=IGC(3,K,1)*T1+IGC(1,K,1)*IN(25)+IGC(2,K,1)*IN(26)
158         48 CONTINUE
159      C
160      C  SECTION 5
161      C
162            MO=MOK(1)
163            DO 49 K=1,8
164            MO=MO+PD(K)*PHV(K)
165         49 CONTINUE
166            PL11=PH(1)
167      C
168      C THE FOLLOWING OUTPUT STATEMENTS ARE OMITTED IN
169      C OPTIMIZATION RUNS.
170      C THE SAME WRITE STATEMENTS APPEAR AT THE END OF EACH
170.5    C AGE GROUP CODE SEGMENT.
172      C
173            WRITE(2,210)Y
174            WRITE(2,207)Z,PH
175            WRITE(2,208)PD,MO
176            WRITE(2,203)
177      C
178      C AGE GROUP 1-12
179      C  SECTION 1
```

```
180       C    STEP 1.1
181       C     FIRST GET A.G. BASELINE POP., THEN USE AS RELEVANT  POP IN XP CALC.
182       C
183               XP(23)=X(23)/(N(8)*(1-MO))
184               N32=N(8)*(1-MO)*12.036
185               DO 50 K=24,26
186               XP(K)=X(K)/N32
187          50   CONTINUE
188       C
189       C    STEP 1.2 AND STEP 1.3
190               DO 52 K=1,2
191               U(K)=SU(K,2)+IUC(1,K,2)*XP(1)+IUC(2,K,2)*XP(22)
192               Y(K)=1.0/(1.0+DEXP(-U(K)))
193          52   CONTINUE
194       C
195       C    STEP 1.4
196       C
197               IN(27)=XP(23)
198               IN(28)=DMIN1(XP(24),Y(1))
199               Y(2)=IN(28)+(1.0-IN(28))*Y(2)
200               IN(29)=DMIN1(XP(25),Y(1))
201               IN(30)=DMIN1(XP(26),Y(4))
202               IN(31)=Y(4)-IN(30)
203       C
204       C   SECTION 2
205       C    STEP 2.1
206       C
207               Z(1)=SZ(1,2)+IZC(1,1,2)*IN(1)+IZC(28,1,2)*IN(28)+IZC(29,
208              11,2)*IN(29)+IZC(30,1,2)*IN(30)+IZC(31,1,2)*IN(31)
209               Z(2)=SZ(2,2)+IZC(1,2,2)*IN(1)
210               Z(3)=SZ(3,2)
211               Z(4)=SZ(4,2)
212               DO 60 K=2,3
213               DO 62 I=20,28
214               Z(K)=Z(K)+IZC(I,K,2)*IN(I)
215          62   CONTINUE
216          60   CONTINUE
217               DO 61 K=2,4
218               Z(K)=Z(K)+IZC(31,K,2)*(IN(31)+IN(30))
219          61   CONTINUE
220       C
221       C    STEP 2.2
222       C
223               DO 65 K=1,4
224               AZ(K)=MAC(K,2)*(PHU(K,2)/(1+DEXP(-Z(K)))+PHL(K,2))
225          65   CONTINUE
226               AZ(1)=AZ(1)+MCC(1)*PL11
227       C
228       C    STEP 2.3
229       C
230               PH(1)=F12*(AZ(1)+MBC(2,1,2)*AZ(2)+MBC(3,1,2)*AZ(3))
231               PH(2)=AZ(2)+MBC(1,2,2)*PH(1)
232               PH(3)=AZ(3)+MBC(1,3,2)*PH(1)
233       C
234       C     ADJUST PH4 FOR DPT & POLIO IMMUNIZATION LEVEL DOMINANCE.
235       C
236               D1=1.-.85*IN(27)
237               PH(4)=D1*AZ(4)
238       C
239       C   SECTION 3
```

```
240      C    STEP 3.1
241      C
242             CALL PHCOM2
243      C
244      C  SECTION 4
245      C    STEP 4.1
246      C
247             PHVSUM=0.0
248             DO 67 K=1,8
249             PHVSUM=PHVSUM+PHV(K)
250        67   CONTINUE
251             WT=PHVSUM*N32
252             XP(27)=X(27)/WT
253             XP(28)=X(28)/WT
254             TXP=XP(27)+XP(28)
255      C
256      C    STEP 4.2
257      C
258             T2=DMIN1(TXP,Y(2))
259             T1=1-T2
260             IN(33)=DMIN1(XP(28),Y(2))
261             IN(32)=T2-IN(33)
262      C
263      C    STEP 4.3
264      C
265             DO 76 K=1,8
266             PD(K)=IGC(3,K,2)*T1+IGC(1,K,2)*IN(32)+IGC(2,K,2)*IN(33)
267        76   CONTINUE
268      C
269      C  SECTION 5
270      C
271             MO1=MOK(2)
272             DO 78 K=1,8
273             MO1=MO1+PD(K)*PHV(K)
274        78   CONTINUE
275             MO=1-(1-MO1)**12.036
276             PL12=PH(1)
277      C
278      C    OUTPUT FOR AGE GROUP 1-12.
279      C
280             WRITE(2,210)Y
281             WRITE(2,207)Z,PH
282             WRITE(2,208)PD,MO
283             WRITE(2,204)
284      C
285      C AGE GROUP 12-60
286      C  SECTION 1
287      C    STEP 1.1
288      C     AGAIN GET A.G. BASELINE POP., THEN USE AS RELEVANT  POP. IN XP CALC.
289      C
290             N33=N32*(1-MO)*4.33
291             DO 80 K=29,30
292             XP(K)=X(K)/N33
293        80   CONTINUE
294      C
295      C    STEP 1.2 AND STEP 1.3
296             DO 82 K=1,2
297             U(K)=SU(K,3)+IUC(1,K,3)*XP(1)+IUC(2,K,3)*XP(22)
298             Y(K)=1.0/(1.0+DEXP(-U(K)))
299        82   CONTINUE
```

```
300      C
301      C    STEP 1.4
302      C
303             IN(34)=DMIN1(XP(29),Y(1))
304             Y(2)=IN(34)+(1.0-IN(34))*Y(2)
305             IN(35)=DMIN1(XP(30),Y(1))
306      C
307      C   SECTION 2
308      C    STEP 2.1
309      C
310             Z(1)=SZ(1,3)+IZC(1,1,3)*IN(1)+IZC(34,1,3)*IN(34)+IZC(35,1,3
311           1)*IN(35)
312             Z(2)=SZ(2,3)+IZC(1,2,3)*IN(1)+IZC(20,2,3)*IN(20)+IZC(21,2,3)
313           1*IN(21)+IZC(22,2,3)*IN(22)+IZC(23,2,3)*IN(23)+IZC(34,2,3)
314           2*IN(34)
315             Z(3)=SZ(3,3)+IZC(22,3,3)*IN(22)+IZC(23,3,3)*IN(23)+IZC(
316           134,3,3)*IN(34)
317             Z(4)=SZ(4,3)+IZC(22,4,3)*IN(22)+IZC(23,4,3)*IN(23)+IZC(3
318           14,4,3)*IN(34)
319      C
320      C    STEP 2.2
321      C
322             DO 97 K=1,4
323             AZ(K)=MAC(K,3)*(PHU(K,3)/(1+DEXP(-Z(K)))+PHL(K,3))
324        97   CONTINUE
325             AZ(1)=AZ(1)+MCC(2)*PL12
326      C    STEP 2.3
327      C
328             F13=1/(1-MBC(2,1,3)*MBC(1,2,3)-MBC(3,1,3)*MBC(1,3,3)-MBC
329           1(3,1,3)*MBC(4,3,3)*MBC(1,4,3)*D1-MBC(4,1,3)*MBC(1,4,3)*D1)
330             PH(1)=AZ(1)+MBC(2,1,3)*AZ(2)+MBC(3,1,3)*AZ(3)+(MBC(3,1,3
331           1)*MBC(4,3,3)+MBC(4,1,3))*AZ(4)*D1
332             PH(1)=PH(1)*F13
333             PH(2)=AZ(2)+MBC(1,2,3)*PH(1)
334             PH(4)=D1*(AZ(4)+MBC(1,4,3)*PH(1))
335             PH(3)=AZ(3)+MBC(1,3,3)*PH(1)+MBC(4,3,3)*PH(4)
336      C
337      C   SECTION 3
338      C    STEP 3.1
339      C
340             CALL PHCOM3
341      C
342      C   SECTION 4
343      C    STEP 4.1
344      C
345             PHVSUM=0.0
346             DO 103 K=1,8
347             PHVSUM=PHVSUM+PHV(K)
348       103   CONTINUE
349             WT=PHVSUM*N33
350             XP(31)=X(31)/WT
351             XP(32)=X(32)/WT
352             TXP=XP(31)+XP(32)
353      C
354      C    STEP 4.2
355      C
356             T2=DMIN1(TXP,Y(2))
357             T1=1-T2
358             IN(37)=DMIN1(XP(32),Y(2))
359             IN(36)=T2-IN(37)
```

```
360       C
361       C   STEP 4.3
362       C
363             DO 109 K=1,8
364             PD(K)=IGC(3,K,3)*T1+IGC(1,K,3)*IN(36)+IGC(2,K,3)*IN(37)
365        109  CONTINUE
366       C
367       C  SECTION 5
368       C
369             MO1=MOK(3)
370             DO 111 K=1,8
371             MO1=MO1+PD(K)*PHV(K)
372        111  CONTINUE
373             MO=1-(1-MO1)**52.14
374       C
375       C   OUTPUT FOR AGE GROUP 12-60.
376       C
377             WRITE(2,206)IN
378             WRITE(2,209)XP
379             WRITE(2,210)Y
380             WRITE(2,207)Z,PH
381             WRITE(2,208)PD,MO
382       C
383       C FINALLY, COMPUTE AND WRITE OUT NOS.
384       C
385             NOS=N33*(1-MO)
386             MOFIN=(NOSUB-NOS)/NOSUB
387             WRITE(2,201)NOS,MOFIN
388       C
389        206  FORMAT(' ','IN :',10F9.5/' ',4X,10F9.5/' ',4X,10F9.5/' ',4X,7F9.5)
390        207  FORMAT(' ',' Z :',4F9.5/' ','PH :',4F9.5)
391        208  FORMAT(' ','PD :',8F9.5/' ','MO :',F9.5)
392        209  FORMAT(' ','XP :',10F9.5/' ',4X,10F9.5/' ',4X,10F9.5/' ',4X,2F9.5)
393        210  FORMAT(' ',' Y :',5F9.5)
394        201  FORMAT('0','NOS:',F8.2/' ','MOFIN:',F6.3)
395        202  FORMAT('-','AGE GROUP 1')
396        203  FORMAT('-','AGE GROUP 2')
397        204  FORMAT('-','AGE GROUP 3')
398             RETURN
399             END
END OF FILE
```

```
1             SUBROUTINE PHCOM1
2       C
3             DIMENSION PH(4),PHV(8),PT(11),PA(11)
4             DIMENSION P2(6),P3(4),MBC(4,4,3)
5       C
6             DOUBLE PRECISION PH,PHV,PT,PA,P2,P3,MBC
7             DOUBLE PRECISION X12,X13,X14,X34
8       C
9             DATA PT/11*0.0/,PA/11*0.0/,P2/6*0.0/,P3/4*0.0/
10      C
11            COMMON /SEC2/ MBC
12            COMMON /SEC3/ PH,PHV
13      C
14      C AGE GROUP 0-1
15      C
16            PT(3)=MBC(1,2,1)*PH(1)
17      C
18            PA(3)=PH(2)-PT(3)
19      C
20            P2(1)=PH(1)*PH(3)
21            P2(2)=PH(1)*PA(3)+PT(3)
22            P2(3)=PH(1)*PH(4)
23            P2(4)=PH(3)*PH(2)
24            P2(5)=PH(3)*PH(4)
25            P2(6)=PH(2)*PH(4)
26            P3(1)=PH(1)*PH(3)*PA(3)+PT(3)*PH(3)
27            P3(2)=PH(1)*PH(3)*PH(4)
28            P3(3)=PH(1)*PA(3)*PH(4)+PT(3)*PH(4)
29            P3(4)=PH(3)*PH(2)*PH(4)
30      C
31            PHV(1)=PH(4)
32            PHV(2)=PH(1)-P2(1)-P2(2)-P2(3)+P3(1)+P3(2)+P3(3)
33            PHV(3)=PH(3)-P2(1)-P2(4)-P2(5)+P3(1)+P3(2)+P3(4)
34            PHV(4)=PH(2)-P2(2)-P2(4)-P2(6)+P3(1)+P3(3)+P3(4)
35            PHV(5)=P2(1)-P3(1)-P3(2)
36            PHV(6)=P2(2)-P3(1)-P3(3)
37            PHV(7)=P2(4)-P3(1)-P3(4)
38            PHV(8)=P3(1)
39            WRITE(2,100) PT,PA,P2,P3,PHV
40            RETURN
41      C
42            ENTRY PHCOM2
43      C
44      C AGE GROUP 1-12
45      C
46            PT(1)=MBC(2,1,2)*PH(2)
47            PT(2)=MBC(3,1,2)*PH(3)
48            PT(3)=MBC(1,2,2)*PH(1)
49            PT(4)=MBC(1,3,2)*PH(1)
50            PT(5)=PT(1)+PT(2)
51      C
52            PA(1)=PH(1)-PT(1)
53            PA(2)=PH(1)-PT(2)
54            PA(3)=PH(2)-PT(3)
55            PA(4)=PH(3)-PT(4)
56            PA(5)=PH(1)-PT(5)
57      C
58            X12=PT(1)+PT(3)-PT(1)*PT(3)
59            X13=PT(2)+PT(4)-PT(2)*PT(4)
```

```
60      C
61              P2(1)=PA(1)*PA(3)+X12
62              P2(2)=PA(2)*PA(4)+X13
63              P2(3)=PH(1)*PH(4)
64              P2(4)=PH(2)*PH(3)
65              P2(5)=PH(2)*PH(4)
66              P2(6)=PH(3)*PH(4)
67      C
68              P3(1)=PA(1)*PA(3)*PA(4)+X12*PA(4)+X13*PA(3)+X12*X13
69              P3(2)=P2(1)*PH(4)
70              P3(3)=P2(2)*PH(4)
71              P3(4)=PH(2)*PH(3)*PH(4)
72      C
73              CALL PHVFIN(PH,P2,P3,PHV)
74              WRITE(2,100) PT,PA,P2,P3,PHV
75              RETURN
76      C
77              ENTRY PHCOM3
78      C AGE GROUP 12-60
79      C
80              PT(1)=MBC(2,1,3)*PH(2)
81              PT(2)=MBC(3,1,3)*PH(3)
82              PT(3)=MBC(4,1,3)*PH(4)
83              PT(4)=MBC(1,2,3)*PH(1)
84              PT(5)=MBC(1,3,3)*PH(1)
85              PT(6)=MBC(4,3,3)*PH(4)
86              PT(7)=MBC(1,4,3)*PH(1)
87              PT(8)=PT(1)+PT(2)
88              PT(9)=PT(1)+PT(3)
89              PT(10)=PT(2)+PT(3)
90              PT(11)=PT(5)+PT(6)
91              X12=PT(1)+PT(4)-PT(1)*PT(4)
92              X13=PT(2)+PT(5)-PT(2)*PT(5)
93              X14=PT(3)+PT(7)-PT(7)*PT(3)
94              X34=PT(6)
95      C
96              PA(1)=PH(1)-PT(1)
97              PA(2)=PH(1)-PT(2)
98              PA(3)=PH(1)-PT(3)
99              PA(4)=PH(2)-PT(4)
100             PA(5)=PH(3)-PT(5)
101             PA(6)=PH(3)-PT(6)
102             PA(7)=PH(4)-PT(7)
103             PA(8)=PH(1)-PT(8)
104             PA(9)=PH(1)-PT(9)
105             PA(10)=PH(1)-PT(10)
106             PA(11)=PH(3)-PT(11)
107     C
108     C
109             P2(1)=X12+PA(1)*PA(4)
110             P2(2)=X13+PA(2)*PA(5)
111             P2(3)=X14+PA(3)*PA(7)
112             P2(4)=PH(2)*PH(3)
113             P2(5)=PH(2)*PH(4)
114             P2(6)=X34
115     C
116             P3(1)=PA(8)*PA(4)*PA(5)+X12*PA(5)+X13*PA(4)+X12*X13
117             P3(2)=PA(9)*PA(4)*PA(7)+X12*PA(7)+X14*PA(4)+X12*X14
118             P3(3)=PA(7)*PA(10)*PA(11)+X13*PA(7)+X14*PA(11)+X34*PA(10)+
119            1X13*X14*(1-X34)+X13*X34*(1-X14)+X14*X34*(1-X13)+X13*X14*X34
```

```
    120            P3(4)=PH(2)*PH(4)*PA(6)+X34*PH(2)
    121       C
    122            CALL PHVFIN(PH,P2,P3,PHV)
    123            WRITE(2,100)PT,PA,P2,P3,PHV
    124            RETURN
    125       100  FORMAT('0','PT :',11F8.5/' ','PA :',11F8.5/' ','P2 :',6F8.5/' ','
    126           13 :',4F8.5/' ','PHV :',8F8.5)
    127            END
END OF FILE
```

```
      1              SUBROUTINE PHVFIN(PH,P2,P3,PHV)
      2        C
      3              DIMENSION PH(4),P2(6),P3(4),PHV(8),A(4)
      4        C
      5              DOUBLE PRECISION PH,P2,P3,PHV,A
      6        C
      7              PHV(1)=PH(1)-P2(1)-P2(2)-P2(3)+P3(1)+P3(2)+P3(3)
      8              PHV(2)=PH(2)-P2(1)-P2(4)-P2(5)+P3(1)+P3(2)+P3(4)
      9              PHV(3)=PH(3)-P2(2)-P2(4)-P2(6)+P3(1)+P3(3)+P3(4)
     10              PHV(4)=PH(4)-P2(3)-P2(5)-P2(6)+P3(2)+P3(3)+P3(4)
     11              PHV(5)=P2(3)
     12              PHV(6)=P2(1)-P3(1)-P3(2)
     13              PHV(7)=P2(2)-P3(1)-P3(4)
     14              A(1)=P2(4)
     15              A(2)=P2(5)-P3(2)-P3(4)
     16              A(3)=P2(6)-P3(3)-P3(4)
     17              PHV(8)=A(1)+A(2)+A(3)
     18              RETURN
     19              END
END OF FILE
```

Index

About the Authors

Howard Barnum is an economist at the Center for Research on Economic Development, University of Michigan. He has served as a consultant for the Organization for Economic Cooperation and Development (Development Center), the U.S. Agency for International Development, and the World Bank. He has worked on development projects concerning not only Colombia but also Bangladesh, Indonesia, and Nepal. Dr. Barnum received his Ph.D. from the University of California, Berkeley.

Robin Barlow is Director of the Center for Research on Economic Development. Previously, he served as a consultant for the U.S. Agency for International Development and the World Bank. Dr. Barlow, who has experience on health development projects in Egypt and Morocco, received his Ph.D. in economics from the University of Michigan.

Luis Fajardo is Director of the Proyecto de Nutricion, Universidad del Valle, Cali, Colombia. He has also taught at Harvard University (Department of Pediatrics) and consulted for the U.S. Agency for International Development and the Pan-American Health Organization. Dr. Fajardo has experience in health and nutrition projects in Colombia, the Dominican Republic, and Zaire. He received his M.D. from the Universidad del Valle and M.S. degrees in biochemistry and metabolism from the Massachusetts Institute of Technology.

Alberto Pradilla is regional nutrition officer with the World Health Organization in New Delhi, India. He has also been associated with the Institute of Nutrition of Central America and Panama, the Universidad del Valle (Department of Pediatrics), the Centro International de Agricultura Tropicale, and Harvard University. He has experience in development projects concerning Bangladesh, Colombia, the Dominican Republic, Guatemala, and India. Dr. Pradilla received his M.D. from the Universidad Nacional in Bogotá.